Surviving Prostate Cancer Without Surgery

Bradley Hennenfent, M.D.

Roseville Books

www.RosevilleBooks.com
www.SurvivingProstateCancerWithoutSurgery.org
www.Hennenfent.com

Copyright

ISBN: 0-9717454-1-2
ISBN 13: 978-0-9717454-1-4

Library of Congress Control Number: 2004096255

Roseville Books
www.RosevilleBooks.com
E-mail: Roseville.Books@gmail.com
Fax: 206-350-1242

To order more books see Amazon.com.

To comment on this book send e-mail to:
Dr.Hennenfent@gmail.com

SurvivingProstateCancerWithoutSurgery.org

10 9 8 7 6 5 4

Other Books by Dr. Hennenfent

The Prostatitis Syndromes: Approaches to Treating Bacterial Prostatitis, Non-Bacterial Prostatitis, Prostatodynia, Benign Prostatic Hyperplasia, Sexual Dysfunction, Bashful Bladder Syndrome, Waking At Night to Urinate, And Possibly Preventing Prostate Cancer. ISBN: 0-9717454-0-4. Published in 1996.

The Prostatitis Syndromes: 2nd Edition: is currently being written and expected to be published in 2010.

Table of Contents

Dedication

This book is dedicated to my uncle, Stephen Arthur Mills, who suffered from prostate cancer; and to my uncle, William "Bud" Gillen, who also suffered from prostate cancer. Both uncles are missed. In addition, I dedicate this book to my other three uncles who have suffered prostate cancer.

Disclaimer

This books deals with adult medical problems and is not suitable for children.

The mention of individuals and organizations within this book does not imply that they endorse this book.

See your own physician if you have any medical problems, including prostate cancer. This book does not replace the need to see a competent and licensed medical physician. The information in this book is for educational purposes only and nothing is fail-safe.

The publisher and authors are not rendering any medical or professional services, nor are they endorsing any of the referenced resources; opinions rendered should not be construed as endorsements. The authors and publishers shall have no liability or responsibility with respect to any harm, loss, or damage, caused by, or alleged to be caused by, or in any way arising from, or alleged to be arising from information contained in this book.

Sensible effort has been made to ensure the accuracy of all statements in this book; however, neither the author nor publisher, or anyone associated with this book promise or guarantee that this information is completely accurate. Because of ongoing research, the accuracy and completeness of the information in this book cannot be guaranteed. Inadvertent technical errors, typographical errors, omissions or inaccuracies may have occurred. Statistical data can be interpreted differently. Readers should rely on their licensed physician, not on any information contained within this book; nothing in this book should be acted upon as a recommendation. This book is an educational resource only.

Dr. Hennenfent does not assume responsibility for any diagnosis or treatment made based on the information in this book or in any of his writings. He is providing information, not diagnosing or treating.

The views of this book are those of Dr. Hennenfent, and do not reflect the views of the non-profit Prostatitis Foundation or its directors.

By purchasing or reading this book, you agree to indemnify and hold harmless Dr. Bradley Hennenfent, Roseville Books, RosevilleBooks.com, SurvivingProstateCancerWithoutSurgery.org, any Hennenfent web site, and any affiliates, agents, employees, freelancers, or volunteers, harmless from and against any and all claims, expenses (including attorney's fees), damages, whether known or unknown, intentional or unintentional.

Quotes

"You may not be able to change the world, but at least you can embarrass the guilty" – Jessica Mitford (1917 – 1996), author of *The American Way of Death.*

"Finally the TRUTH will be told! It's been so frustrating seeing what the urology profession is getting away with and everyone is so ignorant about it and nobody seems to know the difference." – Anonymous (in an e-mail to the author)

Opening Glossary

acini – small sacs inside the prostate that secrete prostatic fluid. Singular is acinus.

BPH – benign prostatic hyperplasia. BPH is a non-cancerous type of growth inside the prostate.

PSA – prostate specific antigen. A protein secreted by normal and cancerous prostate cells. Some say normal is 0 – 4 ug/L.

prostate cancer – prostate cells dividing out of control.

prostatitis – inflammation of the prostate.

radical prostatectomy – radical surgery in which the prostate and seminal vesicles are removed, and nerves, arteries, and veins are severed.

seminal vesicles – storage sacs above and on each side of the prostate that secrete seminal fluid and make up part of the semen.

TRUS – transrectal ultrasound. A type of imaging that uses sound waves to take pictures of the prostate and seminal vesicles.

Preface

I started reading the prostate cancer literature in 1984 after my Uncle Steve suddenly died. It still grieves me that he was undoubtedly killed by his prostate cancer treatment. In total, five of my uncles have suffered prostate cancer.

I became a prostate health activist. By 1995 I had founded the Internet newsgroups: sci.med.prostate.prostatitis, sci.med.prostate.BPH, and sci.med.prostate.cancer. I was one of the original founders of the Prostate Problems Mailing List (PPML). My father and I co-founded the nonprofit Prostatitis Foundation (Prostatitis.org). I also started the Epididymitis Foundation (EpididymitisFoundation.org).

I was talking to patients from all over the world and was inundated with complaints. To put it mildly, men are often dissatisfied with urologists and urology. Because of my Internet activity, I suspect that I have had more access to complaints about urologists than any doctor in history.

I was in a perfect position to look over the shoulders of urologists, see what they do, and criticize them. My experience doing physician quality assurance—critiquing what doctors do—also prepared me for this role.

I wrote a book called *The Prostatitis Syndromes*, donating all proceeds to the nonprofit Prostatitis Foundation. As I wrote a second book, I decided to include prostate cancer.

I wrote too much for one book, so I wrote two books, this one on prostate cancer, and a companion book called, *Prostatitis and BPH*, which focuses on waking up at night to urinate, dribbling, prostatitis, BPH, bashful bladder syndrome, vasectomy, epididymitis, and sexual dysfunction.

Prostate cancer is typically the last of the three major prostate diseases to occur. Usually, during a man's lifetime prostatitis occurs first, then BPH, and finally prostate cancer. If you have prostate cancer, odds are overwhelming you already have prostatitis or BPH. So, to fully understand your prostate, you should also read my other book.

I maintain a website for this book about prostate cancer at <u>SurvivingProstateCancerWithoutSurgery.org</u>.

And one last thing: Thank you! I am very gratified that this book became a best seller for its original distribution company during the book's very first year of publication!

The Big Lie

"If people knew the truth, if there was more—I hate to use the word honesty—but I think people could deal with this disease a little better." - unnamed man in a prostate cancer support group.[1]

Two randomized controlled studies have shown that the radical prostatectomy for prostate cancer does not extend life,[2,3] therefore, you need to know about the growing movement to avoid harmful radical surgery.

And in a third randomized controlled study prostate cancer failed 95% of the time - more on that later!

I believe that most prostate cancer surgery has been a sham. It has been misleadingly advertised and it has been ineffective. Urologists introduced radical prostate surgery without doing the necessary clinical studies. They went for money over science.

---

[1] Unnamed Man as quoted by Anne Barnard. "Men Seek 'The Truth' On Prostate Treatments." *Boston Globe*. January 18th, 2003.

[2] Iversen P, Madsen PO, and Corle DK: Radical prostatectomy versus expectant treatment for early carcinoma of the prostate. Twenty-three year follow-up of a prospective randomized trial. *Scandinavian Journal of Urology and Nephrology*, supplement 1995, Jan 1;172:65-72.

[3] Holmberg L, Bill-Axelson A, Helgesen F, Salo JO, Folmerz P, Haggman M, Andersson SO, Spangberg A, Busch C, Nordling S, Palmgren J, Adami HO, Johansson JE, Norlen BJ: Scandinavian Prostatic Cancer Group Study Number 4. A randomized trial comparing radical prostatectomy with watchful waiting in early prostate cancer. *New England Journal of Medicine*. 2002:Sep 12;347(11):781-789.

In February 1994, Arcadio Arguilez, a 62-year-old carpenter living in California, showed up for an appointment with his urologist, 45-year-old Dr. George Paul Szollar. Arguilez carried a concealed 0.25-caliber handgun. Once inside the doctor's office, he pointed the gun at the doctor's groin, fired once, and fled.

The day before, Arguilez had made a home video in which he described the pain and humiliation he had suffered as a result of the radical prostatectomy that Dr. Szollar had performed on him. According to Arguilez, Dr. Szollar had told him that after the surgery, he would feel "like a young man again." Instead, Arquilez, a husband and father of three, was left feeling like no man at all—impotent, incontinent, and devastated. "The feeling of making love will never be part of my life again," he told the camera. "I'm an android."

"I was in so much pain that I would say, 'Lord, take me, I don't want to live any more,'" Arguilez would admit, his voice cracking.

As he spoke to the camera, Arguilez wore a sign across his chest that read: "For Mankind." It was meant as an explanation of what he planned to do. "I intend to blow his penis and testicles off of him," Arguilez said in the video. "His male parts are going." The single bullet did not quite achieve that goal, but it did reportedly leave Dr. Szollar impotent. For his revenge, Arguilez was sentenced to eleven years in prison.

What would drive a man to such violent rage? Betrayal and loss, a betrayal of trust, a loss of manhood; these emotions are at the heart of how men feel when they put their faith in the medical profession, only to find that the price to be paid for misplaced trust is horrifically high. Not many men who have suffered radical prostatectomies would manifest their rage in such a manner, but over the years, I have met many men who have fantasized about homicide when it comes to their urologists.

The Cure-All that Cures Nothing

A cure is when you take an antibiotic for an infection, the infection clears up, and you return to perfect health. The word *cure* should never be used in the same sentence with the phrase "radical prostatectomy."

The radical prostatectomy is a sacrifice, not a cure. Its rate of sexual dysfunction is a whopping 100 percent. It leaves all men without semen, with a smaller penis, and with diminished or altered orgasms. The bad news doesn't end there. The operation leaves perhaps 60 percent of its victims impotent, 49 percent with some degree of urinary incontinence, and 16 percent with urinary strictures (scarring and blocking of the urinary passage).[4]

All of that—as horrible as it is—might even be worth it to some men if the operation were indeed a life-saver. Unfortunately, controlled scientific evidence shows that the radical prostatectomy is a failure.

The Radical Prostatectomy Mistake

The prostate is intertwined with one's manhood in the most intimate way; it's the fulcrum of male sexuality. This leaves men feeling highly vulnerable during a crisis such as prostate cancer.

Cancer is a vicious blow to begin with. Prostate cancer hits a guy where it really hurts—below the belt! For many men, the knee-jerk reaction after the shock has worn off, is: "Can you cut it out, Doc?"

Unfortunately, when health issues arise, the judgment of men is often poor. Men visit doctors less often than women. They tend to be less well-educated consumers, less critical, less challenging, and less inquisitive. Men have

---

[4] Stanford JL, Feng Z, Hamilton AS, Gilliland FD, Stephenson RA, Eley JW, Albertsen PC, Harlan LC, and Potosky AL: Urinary and Sexual Function After Radical Prostatectomy for Clincially Localized Prostate Cancer: The Prostate Cancer Outcomes Study. JAMA. 2000;283(3):354-360.

not been taught to challenge their doctors and they may not demand a second and third opinion.

Some men take so much pride in being decisive that their rapid decision-making actually works against them. Men sometimes tend to choose the most aggressive form of treatment, because they are naturally inclined to favor action over inaction.

In addition, many men run into a chorus of doctors, who have also been trained—or more precisely, brainwashed, to do the most aggressive thing: radical surgery.

All the urologists in the world aren't worth much if their judgment is based on fundamentally flawed science. When it comes to prostate cancer, there is no statistically valid, randomized controlled scientific evidence, that men with prostate cancer live any longer with surgery than without it. What we do know, with absolute certainty, is that men who undergo surgery are harmed. The radical prostatectomy invariably leaves men weakened, often incontinent, sexually dysfunctional, depressed, and emasculated—in other words, physically and emotionally traumatized. Yet the operations continue with tens of thousands being done every year.

Why would a form of treatment so cruel, so radical, so unproven, be practiced so widely? How could a treatment that is, both medically and morally, the modern equivalent of bloodletting, go unchallenged in such a scientifically enlightened age? The answers are as simple as they are scary.

For one thing, urologists are surgeons, and surgeons are trained to cut. Surgeons make their living by operating, not by referring patients to radiologists, oncologists, or cryosurgeons. As cynical as this may sound, it's a simple fact of life. There are plenty of excuses. Some believe that urologists do not perform unnecessary surgery deliberately, maliciously, or exploitatively, but think it results from an unconscious philosophy and a complex professional culture. Some think that when a surgeon advocates surgery, he may believe in his heart that the cure is in the cut. Certainly, his training has been designed to convince him of this.

I find urologists guilty. Guilty of bad science and false advertising. Guilty of bringing medicine down to the level of the snake oil salesman. Urologists go to medical school and receive the same training that all doctors do. There is no excuse.

You don't have to be a statistician to know that statistics can be easily misrepresented and misinterpreted. Numbers, after all, are no less susceptible to manipulation than are words. And since most people—patients and doctors alike—glaze over when they are confronted by statistical evidence, the truth becomes hard to discern. With regard to prostate cancer and prostatectomies, there are very few people who truly understand the numbers behind the research.

"While the doctor studies," goes an old saying, "the patient dies." When it comes to prostate problems; however, the adage might well be: "While the patient studies, the myths die." It's essential for men to learn about their illness and their options. Prostate cancer is shrouded in misinformation. Sometimes, a falsehood can be so big, so incredible, so threatening, that no one even dares to refute it. Is the epidemic of radical prostate surgery a conspiracy? It's at best an example of misguided medicine. The big lie in this case is the widespread claim that the radical prostatectomy cures prostate cancer, because to date, randomized controlled trials say otherwise.

If knowledge is power, then the right knowledge is empowering. If you, or someone you love, are facing prostate cancer, you have to become your own advocate. It doesn't require going to medical school. It requires mastering the knowledge in this book and other resources. There are at least seven different treatments for prostate cancer. Perhaps your urologist has not taken the time to review all of them with you in detail, or has not explained the pros and cons of each. You cannot rely on your urologist to interpret data for you and help you make the best choice. The only way you can ask the right questions, dispute false claims, make wise decisions, and protect the life you hold dear, is to learn enough to challenge the experts and, in the process, become one yourself.

Most prostate cancer is small and slow-growing. This means that approximately 80 percent of men don't need lifesaving treatment for their prostate cancer because they will die from something else before the cancer kills them. If a surgeon takes 100 men with prostate cancer, performs radical prostatectomies on all of them, and 80 percent of them survive to die from something besides their prostate cancer—nothing has been proven. Yet, false claims are being made that the operation cures 80 percent of men with prostate cancer! In fact, just before writing this passage, I read a reporter's prostate cancer story, in which a well-known urologist fools him into believing an even higher cure rate.

The Bottom Line

Based on the best studies we have today (and we will go over them in detail later), prostate cancer surgery is ineffective. It's no better than a placebo according to one controlled study, and does not extend life according to another controlled study.

Yet, the radical prostatectomy remains the urologists' favorite treatment. I'm deeply outraged by this, and you should be too. The radical prostatectomy has taken its place in medical history, right alongside unnecessary hysterectomies and the frontal lobotomy, as a widely performed operation, with no proven benefit.

You may have seen this scandal hinted about in the *Wall Street Journal* or the *New York Times,* but these newspapers have not yet brought about significant change.

Every time another radical prostatectomy is done it's a sad day indeed, sad for the man who is failed by the medical profession, sad for the doctor who serves as an instrument of that failure, and sad for the society that has come to accept so blithely what can only be described as male genital mutilation.

I believe that all of the other prostate cancer treatments discussed in this book are superior to surgery, either because they are more effective, or because they have fewer side effects. Later in this book, with more evidence, I will tell you how I came to these conclusions.

Most importantly, I am going to tell you, based on the best quality medical studies available, what I would do if I had prostate cancer.

Ron's Story

Ron underwent a routine physical and a PSA (prostate specific antigen) blood test. His PSA was elevated suggesting that cancer was present. Ron meekly said what most men say when frightened by prostate cancer: "Cut it out, doctor."

Within weeks of diagnosis a urologist removed Ron's prostate in an operation called the radical prostatectomy. I saw Ron a year or so later.

"Doctors are complete assholes," Ron greeted me, stopping me in my tracks. This was not the Ron that I knew.

"What happened?" I asked.

Ron turned livid. "I can't feel my penis. I'm totally impotent! I drip urine all day long and have to wear diapers."

"I'm sorry— "

"You can't imagine. I want to kill my urologist. I would rather die than live like this. It's humiliating. I hate . . . I have such rage and hatred. I can't do anything. I pee all over myself. Do you know what my urologist wants to do now?"

"What?"

"More surgery. See they mutilate you. Then they get to do more surgeries to try and reverse the mutilations. It's really a sweet racket they have going."

"I'm sorry."

"And you know the worst part?"

I hesitated and said, "No."

"They didn't even cure my cancer!"

Ron was the epitome of bitterness, hatred, and remorse. Some of it was directed towards me, even though I had nothing to do with his surgery, because I'm a doctor. Ron thought I should have warned him. I would have, if I had known then what I know now.

Ron was never told the truth about the risks of the radical prostatectomy. Even more disturbing, Ron was never told the truth about the lack of proven benefit from the radical prostatectomy. I would come to realize that the information Ron needed to know before having the life-altering operation was never available to him—not in a way that he could understand it. Men desperately need to know the pluses and minuses of prostate cancer treatments. They also need to understand which treatments work best.

Prominent Men with Prostate Cancer

It's important to put a human face on prostate cancer. Thanks to many celebrities who have spoken openly about their own prostate cancer, the disease has come out of the closet and can be talked about in mixed company.

People like Rudolph Giuliani, the former Mayor of New York, are helping to cure prostate cancer, just by discussing it publicly. The road to a cure requires notoriety, publicity, and political clout. Celebrities break down barriers and get research money released.

Naturally, when you are diagnosed with prostate cancer, you want to know what other men have done. Looking at what prominent men have done about their prostate cancer is an admittedly non-scientific way of figuring out what you should do for your prostate cancer. The statistician in me cries foul at such an approach, but it's an approach that men often use.

Some celebrities are intelligent and rich; they have almost unlimited resources for researching what to do. What do such men do?

Mayor Rudolph Giuliani

In April 2000, New York Mayor Rudolph Giuliani dropped out of the senate race against Hillary Clinton because of prostate cancer. He needed time to study his disease.

According to press reports, Giuliani was started on hormone blockade and underwent radioactive seed implantation at Mount Sinai Hospital on September 15,

2000 under local anesthetic. His radiation oncologist was Dr. Richard Stock.

The next day the Mayor walked 24 blocks in the German-American Steuben Parade up Fifth Avenue, something he would never have been able to do after surgery. More importantly to me, the powerful, intelligent mayor of New York, who had access to many of the world's best doctors, did not choose surgery.

Andy Grove, PhD

Who could be more powerful and resourceful than TIME Magazine's 1997 man of the year?

Dr. Andy Grove, Chairman of the Board of Intel Corporation, was diagnosed with prostate cancer in 1994. His tumor was thought to be moderately aggressive. He was offered surgery by a urologist, radiation seed implants by another doctor, and then watchful waiting by a third. He found himself mired in the poor science that surrounds prostate cancer. Using his PhD degree in engineering, Grove went to the data himself, studied it, made charts and graphs of treatment outcomes, and saw multiple specialists for opinions. He read about a man who had a radical prostatectomy and was "bitter." The man had lost his health, job, and marriage.

In 1995, Andy Grove underwent a combination of hormone blockade, high-dose radiation seed implants, and external beam radiation. You can read his autobiographical story in "Taking On Prostate Cancer," the cover story of the May 13, 1996 FORTUNE Magazine. Grove's article has become a classic paper for men with prostate cancer. I highly recommend reading his article. Andy Grove's paper serves to warn men about the poor science behind prostate cancer treatments.

Andy Grove remains well according to press reports. TIME Magazine wrote of him that: ". . . he is a man who coldly eyed a diagnosis of prostate cancer, researched the options and ignored his doctor's advice to pursue his own, so far, successful therapy."[5]

THE LESSON: A powerful, intelligent, scientific man, with many resources, went against urological propaganda and refused the knife. He is so disturbed by the poor science behind prostate cancer treatments that he writes an article about it.

Ed DeHart

Ed DeHart, although not a physician, investigated the controversies surrounding prostate cancer treatment so thoroughly that the editor-in-chief of UROLOGY asked him to write about his experience. DeHart's excellent article, "Reflections of a Prostate Cancer Patient," appeared in that journal in 1996.[6]

THE LESSON: Mr. DeHart, who researched the options so well he is actually published, opted for radiation seed implants over surgery as the treatment for his prostate cancer. I highly recommend that you read Ed DeHart's article.

Thomas L. Walker 1996

Reverend Walker was diagnosed with prostate cancer in 1996 when he was only 46 years old. His book, *Brother to Brother: You Don't Have to Die with Prostate Cancer*, was published in 1998. In his book, the Reverend Walker is encouraged to undergo a radical prostatectomy time after time, despite no controlled scientific study showing that the radical prostatectomy extends life. After much contemplation and prayer, the Reverend chose hormone blockade followed by radiation seed implants.

---

[5] Ramo, JC: A Survivor's Tale. TIME. December 29, 1997.
[6] DeHart, Ed: Relections of a Prostate Cancer Patient. UROLOGY. 1996;48(2):171 - 176

Urologist Edward Ackerman

FORTUNE Magazine reported that urologist Edward Ackerman had radiation seed implants for his prostate cancer in 1995, ironically, after performing the radical prostatectomy on hundreds of his own patients.[7] Several men have pointed this out to me over the years as hypocritical behavior. Certainly, it's enlightening that, when forced to make a choice for himself, the urologist chose not to undergo the radical prostatectomy. However, timing played a role, as Ackerman's group, Winter Park Urology, started doing radiation seed implants about 5 years before Dr. Ackerman's diagnosis. Dr. Ackerman has since retired.

Robert Fine, MD

Dr. Robert Fine, a radiologist, was diagnosed with prostate cancer in 1996. His first PSA test was 2.0 (within the normal range), but his PSA rose to 3.7 over 16 months. No doctor felt any lumps or bumps on his prostate. Nevertheless, Dr. Fine underwent a prostatic biopsy and cancer was discovered.

Dr. Fine, who had access to top doctors and who studied the medical literature, chose radiation seed implants over surgery. He and his wife wrote an important book called, *Prostate Cancer: A Doctor's Personal Triumph.* (1999. Paul S. Eriksson, Publisher.)

Dr. Michael Dorso

Dr. Michael Dorso, a physician, was diagnosed with prostate cancer at age 54. Dr. Dorso has a background in physics, and was in Aerospace medicine for six years before going to work for NASA at their High Speed Flight Research Center at Edwards Air Force Base. He surely has a scientific background!

---

[7] Stipp, David: The Gender Gap in Cancer Research. *Fortune.* May 13, 1996.

In his book, *Seeds of Hope: A Physician's Personal Triumph Over Prostate Cancer*, Dr. Dorso describes choosing radiation seed implants. Importantly to me, he did not choose radical surgery.

Seven Men

I have described seven men to you, including a mayor, a CEO, a reverend, and three physicians who all avoided the radical prostatectomy for prostate cancer. Between them they have published two articles and three books on prostate cancer. All these men chose radiation seed therapy, sometimes combined with other therapies – good choices although not necessarily what I would do, but more about that later. Importantly, powerful and studious men are choosing not to undergo radical surgery! I want to describe one more case to you.

Michael Korda

Michael Korda, Editor-in-Chief at Simon and Schuster Publishing Company, provides an excellent example of how difficult it is for men to learn the statistics of prostate cancer. He wrote about his ordeal in his insightful book, *Man to Man: Surviving Prostate Cancer.*

In his late fifties Korda suffered from symptoms of waking at night to urinate, urgency to urinate, and frequent urination. He would be treated off and on until 1994, when, in his 60s, he had a PSA test, which was elevated.

According to his book, Korda was biopsied without sedation, in fact, without even being given the opportunity to be sedated. In his book, he warns other men that they have a choice about sedation or anesthesia for their biopsies. Korda's first biopsy caused a flare-up of prostatitis. It also missed his prostate cancer. His second biopsy found cancer (Gleason score of 6, PSA = 22).

Korda went to talk to urologist Patrick Walsh about his cancer and pulled medical articles from his briefcase. Korda describes what happened next:

> "Dr. Walsh's geniality vanished instantly. He grabbed the papers out of my hands and flipped through them. 'Who gave you these?' he asked."[8]

Korda was told to forget about the papers or to throw them away. He never got to go over the ten-year survival rates!

Without help from doctors, it's easy to see why men cannot understand the statistics behind prostate cancer therapies.

Korda needed three pints of blood because of his radical prostatectomy, two during surgery, and one post-operatively for a precipitous drop in blood pressure. His post-operative pain machine to drip morphine didn't work, so he received no painkiller during that time despite complaining over and over again about pain.

His quality of life after the operation is problematic. Korda reports in his book that at nine months after surgery he has incontinence "he can live with," and, according to him, has "no erections to speak of..."

I recommend that every man facing prostate cancer read Michael Korda's book for its realistic portrayal of prostate cancer and the radical prostatectomy.

I believe that Michael Korda was never afforded the chance to understand the statistics behind prostate cancer treatments. Don't let this happen to you, read *his* book, read *this* book, talk to other men, and surf the Internet!

---

[8] Korda, Michael. *Man to Man: Surviving Prostate Cancer.* New York: Vintage Books - a Division of Random House, 1997, p. 96. Quoted with signed, written permission.

A Warning about Celebrities

I think many celebrities do the wrong thing. This may be because a lot of celebrities do not have a scientific bent and rely on their doctors to tell them what to do.

Some people feel that many celebrity prostate cancer patients have avoided talking about what men really want to know about—issues like impotence, incontinence, and other side effects—especially after radical surgery. Indeed, what you often see is celebrities playing the role of "hero" for having undergone prostate surgery, instead of talking about the intimate side effects that other men really want to know about.

Many women feel left out in the cold. Prostate cancer treatment often devastates the sex lives and physical intimacy that couples normally enjoy. Women sometimes feel betrayed that no one tells them what prostate cancer or its treatment is going to do to their relationship with their lover. One woman suggested to me that we have enough heroes: it's time for the truth; it's time for full disclosure.

Conclusion

I have observed a pattern, which is that well-educated men with more time, money, and resources, are avoiding the radical prostatectomy, while the urologist often rushes John Q. Public to surgery.

Well-educated men are writing books and articles about their prostate cancer experience, because when they research on their own, they often end up defying urologists' recommendations for surgery. Standing up against such pressure spurs them to write about why they did it.

You need to know the data behind the decision-making. Before this book is over, we will go to the data ourselves.

What is Prostate Cancer?

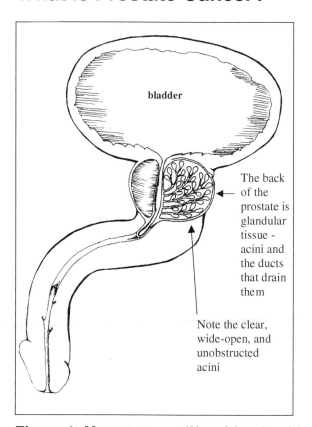

bladder

The back of the prostate is glandular tissue - acini and the ducts that drain them

Note the clear, wide-open, and unobstructed acini

Figure 1. Men start out life with a healthy prostate.

Prostate cancer occurs when prostate cells multiply and grow out of control, instead of dying off after a normal lifespan. Prostate cancer cells, like all cancer cells, are immortal—they don't die when their time is up.

Prostate cancer cells form a tumor. Sometimes the tumor spreads outside the prostate, extending regionally, to affect nearby organs. At other times, prostate cancer cells break away and travel (metastasize) to other parts of the body, such as the bones or lungs, where they start new tumors.

Importantly, the local tumor inside the prostate almost never kills anyone. With prostate cancer, it's the metastases that kill men. You should pay more attention to treating any possible spread of prostate cancer, than to simply killing the tumor inside your prostate.

For example, the more aggressive forms of prostate cancer are infamous for getting into the lower spine and pressing on the spinal cord, which can paralyze a man from the waist down and eventually kill him.

Controversial

Prostate cancer is controversial. At the highest levels of academic medicine, doctors can't agree on what causes it, how to diagnose it, or how to treat it.

Prostate Cancer is Common

You are almost certain to get prostate cancer; all you have to do is live long enough for it to erupt inside of you. As the pie chart shows, by the time men are over 50 years old, forty percent already have prostate cancer.

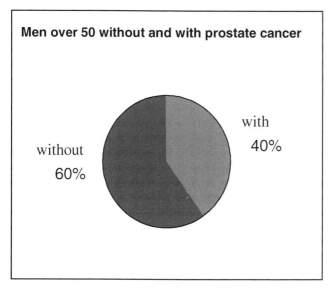

Men over 50 without and with prostate cancer

without
60%

with
40%

Figure 2. Forty percent of men over fifty years of age have prostate cancer.[9]

Prostate cancer is the most commonly diagnosed cancer among men in the United States and is the second most common cause of all cancer deaths in men, behind lung cancer. Microscopic prostate cancer is found in 20 percent of all men by age 30 and in nearly 100 percent of men by age 90.

Since 1989 the incidence of prostate cancer has risen dramatically. Many suspect that this epidemic was largely due to the ability of the PSA (prostate specific antigen) test to pick up never before detected cancers. In 2003, according to the Centers for Disease Control, 220,900 new cases of prostate cancer were diagnosed and 28,900 men died from prostate cancer.

---

[9] Stamey, Thomas: Prostate Cancer: Who Should Be Treated? April 1994. Accessed July 18, 2004 at: www.prostatepointers.org/prostate/stamey/stamey.html.

Age of Discovery

Until recently, prostate cancer usually was diagnosed in men between 60 to 80 years old. In fact, prostate cancer used to be diagnosed in men at an average age of 72, but because of the PSA test, prostate cancer is being found in younger men. A survey of 1000 members of Us TOO International (a prostate cancer support group) found that about half of them were diagnosed between the ages of sixty and sixty-nine,[10] but the PSA test is also finding prostate cancer in men who are in their 30s, 40s, and 50s.

Low Death Rate

Prostate cancer has a very low death rate compared to other cancers. Only three percent of all men in the USA die from prostate cancer, despite the high percentage of men who have it.

Instead of all men in the USA, let's look at only men who actually have prostate cancer. Of all men with prostate cancer in the USA, diagnosed or not, only 7.5 percent will die from it.[11] That's a very low death rate for a cancer!

But your risk of death is higher once you are diagnosed with prostate cancer. Of all the men with prostate cancer, only a percentage of them actually get diagnosed as having it. Once you are diagnosed you enter an even smaller pool of men. Your risk of death could range from 4 percent to 87 percent depending on the type and size of your prostate cancer.[12] In many places throughout this book we will review studies and address these odds. In addition, you

---

[10] Louis Harris and Associates: Perspectives on Prostate Cancer Treatments: Awareness, Attitudes, and Relationnships. Conducted for Us TOO International, Inc. 1995.

[11] Stamey, Thomas: Prostate Cancer: Who Should Be Treated? April 1994. Accessed July 18, 2004 at: www.prostatepointers.org/prostate/stamey/stamey.html.

[12] Albertsen PC, Hanley JA, Gleason DF, and Barry MJ: Competing Risk Analysis of Men Aged 55 to 74 Years at Diagnosis Managed Conservatively for Clinically Localized Prostate Cancer. JAMA 1998;280(11):975-980.

are responsible for determining your own risk, based on your cancer's characteristics, using resources in this book and elsewhere.

Most Prostate Cancer is Slow-Growing

Prostate cancer is unlike any other cancer. What makes prostate cancer so unique is that most prostate cancer is *slow-growing.* As a consequence, most men with prostate cancer will die with it, not from it.

Many kinds of cancer will double in size in a matter of months, but not prostate cancer. Of men diagnosed with prostate cancer, 80 percent of them have cancers that take four or five years to double in size. This is remarkable, as almost no other cancer is so slow-growing.

It's the more aggressive 20 percent of prostate cancer that doctors and patients worry about; it's the kind that either causes symptoms or kills.

In men with prostate cancer, 7.5 percent grows rapidly enough to kill, while 12.5 percent of prostate cancers become large enough to cause symptoms. That adds up to the 20 percent of prostate cancer that is aggressive enough to kill or cause symptoms.[13]

THE OBVIOUS POINT: 80 percent of prostate cancer doesn't grow quickly enough to kill or cause symptoms, yet most men seem sure that they are in the unlucky 20 percent when they are told they have prostate cancer.

Unfortunately, current medical technology is not very effective at distinguishing fast-growing from slow-growing prostate cancer. Consequently, physicians often resort to treating every man with prostate cancer as though they will die from it, although the vast majority of them are not in danger of dying. When this approach is undertaken, about

---

[13] Stamey TA, Freiha FS, McNeal JE, Redwine EA, Whittemore AS, Schmid HP: Localized prostate cancer. Relationship of tumor volume to clinical significance for treatment of prostate cancer. *Cancer* 1993:Feb 1;71(3 Suppl):933-938.

80 percent of men with prostate cancer will receive unnecessary treatment and suffer needless side effects.

Most Prostate Cancer is Small

Most prostate cancer tumors are between the size of a pellet from a BB gun and a small pea. Urologist Thomas Stamey and his colleagues at Stanford are pioneers in relating the size of prostate cancer tumors to the cancer's aggressiveness. Their work suggests that 80 percent of all prostate cancers are less than one-fourth inch in diameter. In metric terms, 80 percent of prostate cancers are thought to be smaller than 0.5 ml and probably never reach a big enough size to cause symptoms.[14]

If your BB- or pea-sized tumor only doubles in size every five years, and like most men you are in your sixties when diagnosed, you will probably die of some other problem before your prostate cancer can kill you. The majority of the time, prostate cancer is tiny, slow-growing, and doesn't kill. It's the exceptions to this rule that cause all the trouble.

Prostate cancer pathologist, Dr. John McNeal, reported in 1993 that metastatic cancer only occurred with prostate cancer larger than 4 ccs in volume that contained Grade 4 or higher Gleason scores.[15] Four cc of volume is slightly less than a teaspoon. Take a teaspoon of water and look at it in a cup; most prostate cancer up to that size is not lethal. The study suggests that you need at least that volume of prostate cancer inside you with a Gleason score above 4 to get metastatic prostate cancer—although there are probably exceptions. Tumors larger than 12 cc in volume—slightly less than a tablespoon—tend to always be lethal. The general rule is the greater the volume of prostate

---

[14] Stamey TA, Freiha FS, McNeal JE, Redwine EA, Whittemore AS, Schmid HP: Localized prostate cancer. Relationship of tumor volume to clinical significance for treatment of prostate cancer. *Cancer.* 1993;Feb 1;71(3 Suppl):933-938.

[15] McNeal JE: Prostatic microcarcinomas in relation to cancer origin and the evolution to clinical cancer. *Cancer.* 1993;71(3 suppl):984-991.

cancer inside you the more likely metastasis is to occur and the more likely that death will occur.

White American men have a life expectancy of 74.3 years, and black American men have a life expectancy of 67.2 years. Many urological papers recommend that few men over 70 years of age should have aggressive treatment for asymptomatic prostate cancer because so many of them die of other causes before their prostate cancer has time to become large enough to trouble them. Small cancers can be harbored for years, or decades, before they grow big enough to cause you any trouble, so one of the first things you will want to know when diagnosed with prostate cancer is the size of the tumor inside you.

A significant percentage of prostatic cancers removed at surgery are less than one-fourth inch in size—so small that they would probably never have hurt the men who underwent the surgery, because the men would have died from other causes before their cancer became lethal.

The larger the cancer, however, the more likely it is to be aggressive and dangerous. Fortunately, the larger prostate cancers are rare, although it is hard for men to keep this in perspective.

TO REPEAT: As urologist Thomas Stamey has written, in the United States only 3 percent of the male population dies from prostate cancer. If we only look at men who have prostate cancer as our denominator, only 7.5 percent of men with prostate cancer die from it. NEVER FORGET THESE TWO NUMBERS, because the odds are with you, not against you.

While the odds of prostate cancer killing a man are small, the fact that prostate cancer afflicts so much of the male population means that a lot of men will die from it. It's been estimated that 3 million men living today in the United States will eventually die from prostate cancer.

All this presents men with a dilemma: since most prostate cancer grows slowly, most men with it would be better off if doctors left them alone. Men have to ask themselves if treatments such as surgery, radiation, cryoablation, or hormone blockade therapy are an improvement over doing nothing.

Unfortunately, when it comes to prostate cancer, everything is in shades of gray. Some would suggest doing nothing, with good reason, because prostate cancer treatments have serious side effects. Meanwhile, the probability of curing fast-growing prostate cancer is problematic, because it's unclear if doctors can detect it before it has metastasized. Prostate cancer is not like appendicitis, where you become ill, have an operation, and then are cured. Prostate cancer treatments cause damage.

THUS THE TRADGEDY: If doctors do nothing, approximately 80 percent of men diagnosed with prostate cancer will do fine. If doctors aggressively treat all men with prostate cancer to get at the 20 percent who really need treatment, all the men are damaged—sometimes very seriously damaged—for the rest of their lives.

Prostate Cancer Symptoms

According to conventional wisdom, most prostate cancer is silent; it does not cause men any symptoms. When prostate cancer does cause symptoms, they include difficulties with urination, such as waking at night to urinate (nocturia), dribbling after urination, frequency, urgency, hesitancy, weak stream, or incomplete emptying of the bladder. Other symptoms may include low back pain, weight loss, loss of energy, and loss of appetite. Prostate cancer can cause sexual dysfunction, including impotence, fewer erections and less hard erections, lower semen volume, bloody semen, and more down time between erections.

Many men with prostate cancer are diagnosed with, or have all the symptoms of prostatitis or benign prostatic hyperplasia (BPH), before their prostate cancer is diagnosed.

It is one of the lessons of this book that virtually all men with prostate cancer should be tested for prostatitis and BPH. Treating prostatitis and BPH may cause your PSA level to go down and spare you from undergoing an unnecessary biopsy. In addition, treating prostatitis may cure your symptoms and turn you from seeking aggressive treatment into someone who is willing to watch and wait, perhaps for the rest of your life, as you look into other options for treatment.

See my previously published book, *The Prostatitis Syndromes*, or my soon to be published book, *Prostatitis and BPH*, for more information about treating prostatitis and BPH and avoiding unnecessary biopsies.

What Causes Prostate Cancer?

What causes prostate cancer? What starts the whole process where normal cells suddenly grow out of control? Interestingly, the scientific community has some pretty strong prejudices about what causes prostate cancer. Some think that prostate cancer comes from something within the human body—bad genes—while others think that prostate cancer comes from something outside the body—carcinogens.

Genes

Some researchers think that the different rates of prostate cancer among different ethnic groups are evidence that prostate cancer has a genetic component. African-American men have the highest rate of prostate cancer in the world, while white men in the United States and Swedish men are close behind them. In contrast, Japanese and Chinese men are unlikely to die from prostate cancer.

Doctors disagree about how much of prostate cancer is hereditary; estimates range from 3 to 40 percent. In a small minority of all men with prostate cancer a gene has been identified that appears to be a "prostate cancer" gene. But most experts agree that it appears unlikely that genes account for all the different rates of prostate cancer. We may have bad genes inside of us, oncogenes, which will turn a cell cancerous, but something probably has to trigger them, so most believe that environmental factors must play an important role in causing cancer.

Environment and Occupation

Lack of sunlight may be related to prostate cancer. People in the northern latitudes seem to be at a greater risk for prostate cancer than the general population.

Farmers have a higher risk of prostate cancer according to some studies, and some suspect exposure to pesticides as the culprit. Or, it may be that riding machinery tends to plug up farmers' prostates, causing cancer down the road.

One study found an association between smoking and prostate cancer.[16] This is hardly surprising since smoking is linked to so many kinds of cancer.

There is suspicion about Agent Orange causing prostate cancer. At least one organization has suggested that anyone who served in Vietnam who was exposed to Agent Orange should undergo prostate cancer screening.

Anabolic steroids are prescription drugs that bodybuilders and other athletes sometimes take illicitly to increase their muscle mass. Taking anabolic steroids is thought to increase the risk of getting prostate cancer.

The element cadmium has been associated with prostate cancer. Cadmium is used in alloys, newspaper printing, dental amalgams, nickel-cadmium storage batteries, and nuclear reactor shields, among other things. Welders and those who solder electrical components together may be exposed to cadmium.

One study estimated that 12 percent of prostate cancer might be due to environmental exposure from working in certain occupations.[17]

There is evidence that a high fat diet contributes to prostate cancer. Some studies have even found a relationship between high cholesterol and prostate cancer.

---

[16] Coughlin S, Neaton J, Sengupta A: Cigarette smoking as a predictor of death from prostate cancer in 348,874 men screened for the Multiple Risk Factor Intervention Trial. *American Journal of Epidemiology.* 1996;143(10):1002-6.

[17] Kristan Aronson et al.: Occupational risk factors for prostate cancer: results from a case-control study in Monteal, Quebec, Canada, *Mediconsult.com Limited.*

Anatomy

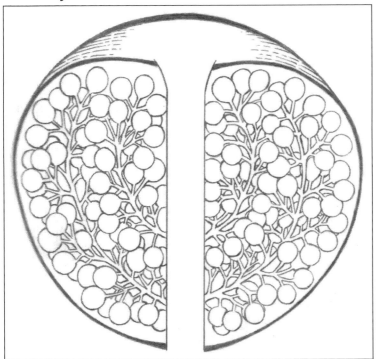

Figure 3. The prostate is separated into right and left halves by the urethra. Each side of the prostate is full of acini, which are sacs that secrete prostatic fluid. This is a concept drawing; the ducts and acini are actually microscopic in size. (Artist: Ramie Balbuena)

As the drawing shows, your prostate is filled with glands. The glands consist of little sacs that produce prostatic fluid and then drain into ducts. Each side of your prostate looks like a bunch of grapes, with the grapes being the acini (sacs), and the stems being the ducts. Everything leads into the urethra and then flows down and out the penis.

Obstruction

From looking under the microscope, I believe that obstruction of the prostate is one of the earliest things to go wrong with men. This occurs in any of the thousands of acini that men have, and may be silent, thus men are often unaware of the problem.

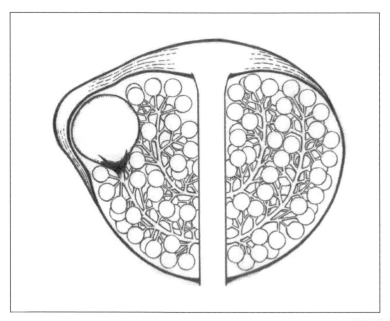

Figure 4. The acinus has blown up like a balloon because the duct leading to it has become obstructed. It's so big that it distorts the prostate. (Artist: Ramie Balbuena)

Inflammation

Obstruction and inflammation of the prostate go together. When an acinus becomes obstructed, white blood cells flock to fight whatever is trapped inside. The inflammation often becomes chronic, and that is why so many men have pus in their prostates. This is disturbing, because we know that chronic inflammation and cancer are strongly associated.

That little sac inside your prostate may be full of pus for decades. Dr. John Polacheck of the Tucson Prostatitis Clinic and pathologist Dr. Edwardo Vega have shown me photomicrographs of what such pus looks like under the microscope. They have named the finding prostatic inflammatory aggregates (PIAs). Dr. Antonio Espinosa Feliciano, Jr., of the Manila Genitourinary Clinic, has shown me this finding as well. I've also seen PIAs in slides presented at medical conferences where the presenters did not know what they had.

Urine

Urine refluxes into the prostate. By old age, virtually all men have "prostate stones" composed of crystallized urine inside them. Perhaps early in a man's life urine refluxes (flows backwards) into his prostate, setting up chemical irritation followed by obstruction of acini.

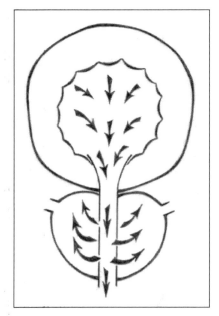

Figure 5. As urine flows from the bladder down through the prostate, it sometimes refluxes into the prostate where it does not belong. (Artist: Ramie Balbuena)

Semen

Semen refluxes into the prostate. We know this because sperm can sometimes be found inside the prostate when deceased men are autopsied.

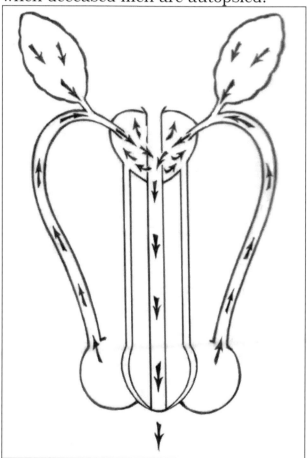

Figure 6. Semen refluxes into the prostate. Semen consists of sperm from the testicles, the seminal fluid from the seminal vesicles, and the prostatic fluid. (Artist: Ramie Balbuena)

Semen suppresses the immune system. This weakens our prostate's defenses, and may trigger prostatitis, prostate enlargement, or prostate cancer.

One researcher demonstrated, back in 1978, that injecting sperm into rat prostates produced prostate cancer in those animals.[18]

One urologist wrote a unique book, *The Other Guy's Sperm: The Cause of Cancers and Other Diseases*,[19] in which he blames sperm for any number of cancers and illnesses. If sperm sometimes play a role in cancer formation by getting into the wrong place it could help to explain the abnormal chromosome count (aneuploidy) often seen in the more aggressive kinds of prostate cancer.

Bacteria and Viruses

Bacteria get inside the prostate. There are hundreds of studies that have found bacteria inside the prostate. Bacteria are found in men with symptoms, but also in supposedly "healthy" men.

Viruses also get into the prostate. In fact, human papilloma virus (HPV) has been associated with prostate cancer in some studies.

Bags Sitting Inside

Carcinogens may be concentrated inside the prostate. Animal studies have shown that generating prostatic fluid concentrates products from the blood stream, including carcinogens, hundreds of times.

So when your prostate is plugged up, it might contain semen, urine, bacteria, viruses, and carcinogens. Polluted sacs of cancer causing ingredients may be festering inside your prostate for decades. Do we then have a situation that will turn into prostate cancer years later? I think this is a rich cancer-causing environment!

---

[18] Stein-Werblowsky R: On the Etiology of Cancer of the Prostate. *European Urology*. 1978;4:370-373.

[19] Tyler DE: *The Other Guy's Sperm: The Cause of Cancers and Other Diseases*. Ontario: Discovery Books, 1994.

Dr. H. Hale Harvey's Hypothesis

One of the most intriguing theories about what may cause prostate cancer comes from epidemiologist H. Hale Harvey, MD, PhD, MPH. The well-credentialed Dr. Harvey believes that fat plugging up the prostate's arteries (atherosclerosis) leads to cell death in the prostate. This causes surviving cells to release growth signals. These growth signals stimulate benign prostatic hyperplasia (BPH) to occur. BPH, which is a benign tumor, obstructs prostatic ducts causing the acini behind the obstruction to blow up like balloons. The increased pressure distorts the cells lining the acini, turning them into deformed cells with greater growth potential (doctors have a fancy phrase for this calling it prostatic intraepithelial neoplasia, or PIN). These new cells try to overcome the rising pressure within the blocked acini.

First, low-grade PIN occurs, and as the blockage continues and pressure increases, high-grade PIN occurs. Finally the acini burst and the PIN cells are exploded into the tissue, called stroma, between the acini. The PIN cells, now in the wrong place, are no longer inhibited from multiplying out of control as they would be in their normal environment. Prostate cancer begins as the cells divide over and over again.

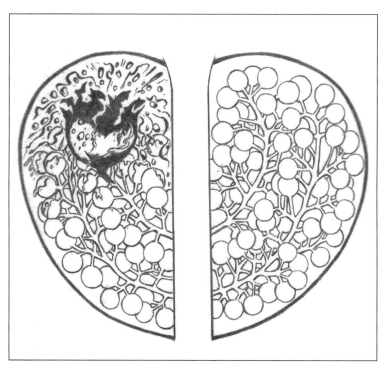

Figure 7. When the obstructed acinus bursts it sends cells into the body of the prostate where they are not supposed to be. Those cells may then turn into prostate cancer. (Artist: Ramie Balbuena)

Dr. Harvey's hypothesis of fat plugging up the prostate's arteries, cell death, production of growth stimulating factors, the occurrence of BPH causing obstruction, distended acini, and abnormal cells bursting into the stroma, explains a lot about prostate cancer.

Harvey's theory explains why a high fat diet might be associated with prostate cancer, why genetic mutations are not necessary for the formation of prostate cancer, and why prostate cancer looks the way it does under the microscope.[20]

---

[20] H. Hale Harvey: A Unifying Hypothesis that Links Benign Prostatic Hyperplasia and Prostatic Intraepithelial Neoplasia with Prostate Cancer. *Pathology Research and Practice.* 1995;191:924-934.

Dr. Harvey believes that regular sexual activity is important to keep the prostatic acini unblocked and believes that the interruption of sexual activity for a period of time during a man's life is probably a risk factor for prostate cancer. He feels that there is a strong argument that prostatitis is a cause of some cases of prostate cancer. Dr. Harvey has practiced self-prostatic massage for years and believes that it would be wise for all men to do so.[21] See my other books, *The Prostatitis Syndromes*, or *Prostatitis and BPH*, for details about prostatic massage and instructions on how to do it.

Two Studies on Sex

Two studies support the idea that it's bad to let your prostate stagnate. An Australian study compared the ejaculation history of 1,079 men with prostate cancer to 1,259 healthy men. The study concluded that men who ejaculated frequently in their twenties and thirties were less likely to get prostate cancer later in life. In fact, those who ejaculated more than 5 times per week in their 20s were significantly less likely to get prostate cancer later.[22] The study also found that masturbation was more protective than sexual intercourse and suggested that the reason might be because infections associated with intercourse do not occur with masturbation.

A study done in the United States also found increased sexual activity to be protective against prostate cancer. The study of 29,000 men, from 1992 to 2000,

---

[21] H. Hale Harvey: Telephone interview with the author. April 2, 1999. Paraphrased with signed, written permission.

[22] Giles GG, Severi G, English DR, McCredie MR, Borland R, Boyle P, Hopper JL: Sexual factors and prostate cancer. *BJU International.* 2003 Aug;92(3):211-216.

showed that those who ejaculated the most were one-third less likely to get prostate cancer.[23]

These studies lead to speculation on why frequent ejaculation might prevent prostate cancer. Researchers have suggested that: ejaculation keeps all the prostatic acini clean from blockage; ejaculation may prevent carcinogens from building up inside the prostate; that frequent ejaculation prevents the build-up of tiny calcifications inside the prostate, which have been associated with prostate cancer; that stagnant prostatic fluid suppresses the prostate's ability to fight cancer cells; and that ejaculation helps the prostate cells mature more quickly which makes them less likely to turn cancerous.

Massage Study

I'd like to see a study subjecting men to repetitive, prostatic massage as prevention for prostate cancer. We need to empty men's prostates of the little "bags of carcinogens and germs" that they have inside of them as a result of their prostates getting plugged up—bags of debris that ejaculation alone cannot expel. In one arm of the study would be men whose prostates were kept free of pus and bacteria with repetitive massage and antibiotics; we wouldn't let their acini swell up from obstruction and explode into the stroma of their prostates. In the other arm of the study a group of men would be allowed to follow the natural course of events. Which group would suffer more prostatitis, BPH and prostate cancer?

Breast cancer

I have noticed important analogies about infection and breast cancer, which can be related to prostate cancer.

---

[23] Leitzmann, M.F., Platz, E.A., Stampfer, M.J., Willett, W.C., and Giovannucci, E. Ejaculation frequency and subsequent risk of Prostate Cancer. JAMA. 2004 Apr 7;291(13):1578-86.

Epstein-Barr virus has been associated with breast cancer. In fact there is a region in Africa known as the "breast cancer belt" where the Epstein Barr virus is common. Virologists have shown the presence of Epstein-Barr viral DNA in women with breast cancer and its absence in women without the disease.[24] This virus may make breast cancer look hereditary by being passed from mother to daughter, where the virus lays dormant until the hormones of puberty ignite it.

Which brings me to another point about how it is healthy for organs like the breast and prostate to drain properly. It's been suggested that troubles with the lymphatic system may play a role in breast cancer. Sydney Ross Singer and Soma Grismaijer, in their book, *Dressed to Kill*, talk about how wearing a brassiere may pinch off lymphatic drainage of the breast, and thus predispose women to get breast cancer. They note the very interesting and alarming statistic that the breast cancer incidence rate in non-bra wearing cultures is only 1 in 168 women, while the breast cancer rate in bra wearing countries like the US, Japan, and Western Europe 1 in 8.

Some studies have indicated that women with breast cancer have histories of wearing tighter bras and wearing bras for more hours per day than women without breast cancer. There appears to be a link between constricting the breasts and breast cancer.

Why might there be such a link? Bras apply pressure to the breasts and constrict the normal drainage of the lymphatic system. The lymphatic system consists of delicate vessels that drain all the body's tissues of toxins, cell debris, viruses, and bacteria. Squeezing the lymphatic system and blocking it allows toxins to build up. Many researchers have advised women not to wear a bra to sleep and not to wear constrictive bras. And many suggest decreasing the number of hours per day that a bra is worn.

---

[24] Fackelmann, Kathleen: A Versatile Virus, Epstein-Barr virus displays a few new malignant tricks. *Science News*: 1995;147(7):104-105.

Men have an analogous situation with their prostate. Many men wear pants and a belt and spend all day, bent over, sitting at a desk. Men are literally squeezing their prostates all day long at work and while driving their cars. Seat cushions often push up directly on the prostate. Our lifestyles probably compromise the lymphatic drainage of our prostates and allow toxins to build up inside them.

Conclusion

I think it's time to do a study, based on these theories, to see if keeping prostates clean of obstruction, debris, and infection, can prevent prostate cancer.

Prostatitis and Prostate Cancer

Prostatitis means pus in the prostate. Pus is the layman's term for white blood cells. All the situations described in the last chapter, reflux of semen, urine, bacteria, viruses, and obstruction of the prostate result in prostatitis. You may be surprised to learn, however, that what actually causes prostatitis in the majority of men is a worldwide controversy.

There are three basic diseases of the prostate, prostatitis, BPH (benign prostatic hyperplasia), and prostate cancer. Typically, during a man's lifetime, prostatitis occurs first, then BPH, and then prostate cancer.

Prostatitis can be silent or symptomatic. You can have pus in your prostate and not know about it; that's silent prostatitis.

When prostatitis causes symptoms, it causes dribbling, waking at night to urinate, frequency, pain, and sexual dysfunction.

In men with symptomatic prostatitis, urologists say about 5 percent of prostatitis is bacterial. Urologists are still arguing about the cause of prostatitis in the other 95 percent of men with symptoms. Furthermore, the cause of silent prostatitis remains unknown.

One study found a 30 percent rate of purulent (pus filled) prostatic secretions in young military recruits; they had silent prostatitis.[25] Do these, supposedly healthy men with pus in their prostates in their late teens and 20s, end up getting BPH or prostate cancer at age 60, 70, or 80? Since no one knows what causes most prostatitis, and since

[25] Schwartz: *The Principles of Surgery*. New York: McGraw-Hill, 1979.

the military men in the study weren't followed over time, no one knows whether prostatitis leads to BPH or prostate cancer.

Some researchers suspect that a microbe or microbes will be found that causes prostatitis and also triggers prostate cancer. I expect that a percentage of prostate cancer will eventually be explained by this mechanism. Certainly the proper studies need to be done.

Interestingly, one of the few studies ever done on the issue did show an increased risk of prostate cancer in men with symptomatic prostatitis.[26]

Urologist Ronald Wheeler says:

> "In my opinion, prostatitis resolution holds the key to the future of prostate cancer resolution."[27]

Pathologist Russell L. Kershmann, MD, notes that prostatitis begins in the periphery of the prostate early in life, and prostate cancer occurs in the same location decades later. This suggests that prostatitis may cause prostate cancer.[28]

Urologist Richard Alexander, testifying before congress, said:

> ". . . could chronic inflammation be a cause of prostatic cancer, the most common cancer of men in the United States, or a cause of benign prostatic enlargement? What major

---

[26] Nakarta S: Study of risk factors for prostatic cancer. *Hinyokika Kiyo.* 1993;39(11):1017-1024.

[27] Wheeler Ron: The Incidence of Prostatitis in Men with Voiding Symptoms. *PAACT Communcator.* Sunday March 12th, 2000.

[28] Kerschmann RL: Inflammatory Lesions of the Prostate. A lecture delivered at the Twelfth Annual Current Issues in Anatomic Pathology Meeting. San Francisco. May 23 - 25. 1996. Available at: http://kersch.ucsf.edu/Prostate.Lecture/Prostatitis.html. Quoted with signed, written permission.

and fundamental discovery about the etiology of these common prostate conditions remains hidden because no funds are available for studies of prostatic inflammation?"[29]

Scientist Richard J. Ablin says:

"One of the aspects that's completely overlooked in regards to subsequent diseases of the prostate is prostatitis. There is some suggestion that prostatitis contributes to BPH or prostate cancer, and/or that some change in the microenvironment of the prostate sets up all three diseases."[30]

It only makes sense that what triggers prostate cancer should be found in the gland decades earlier and prostatitis is there! The cause of prostate cancer has no clear cause according to conventional wisdom, yet the medical community is ignoring the most likely cause of prostate cancer—chronic prostatitis. And, I don't mean just symptomatic prostatitis; I include the almost always present, but silent prostatitis as well.

Do Microorganisms cause Prostate Cancer?

We need to take a very hard look at the germs stuck inside blocked-up prostates. Chronic infection is know to be related to at least nine kinds of cancer, yet this possibility is not being aggressively investigated for prostate cancer.

Did you know that it's now believed that the bacteria that causes ulcers, *Helicobacter pylori*, also causes stomach

---

[29] Alexander, Richard: Testimony on behalf of the Prostatitis Foundation to the Subcommittee on Labor, health and Human Services, Education and Related Agencies. April 24, 1997.

[30] Ablin, Richard J: Telephone conversation with the author, December 30th, 1998. Quoted with signed, written permission.

cancer? Why couldn't the same kind of thing be going on inside the prostate?

Different germs getting into the prostate could explain many of the variations seen in prostate cancer. The increased incidence of prostate cancer in African-American men could be due to a particular microbe endemic to that population, as could be the increased incidence of prostate cancer in Swedish men. The fact that Japanese men have a lower rate of clinically significant prostate cancer could be due to their microbial flora (naturally occurring bacteria that they carry inside them), which, when altered by living in the United States, raises their risk of prostate cancer to USA levels.

Study the Tissue

We have a situation where doctors are taking out prostatic tissue from hundreds of thousands of men each year and we could be studying all this tissue, but we are not doing so to my satisfaction.

We can make great progress in proving or disproving whether germs cause prostate cancer in a few years. We can use DNA technology to completely map out the microbial presence in normal prostates, prostates with prostatitis, enlarged prostates, and cancerous prostates.

The only way to be sure if "silent prostatitis," where men are unaware that they have it, or "symptomatic prostatitis" causes prostate cancer is to first find out what is causing prostatitis and then compare men at different ages, or to follow men over their entire lifetimes.

For all we know, 100 different microbes could be causing the prostatitis lesion in men, and perhaps one or two of these could be triggers for prostate cancer. Even "normal bacterial flora," if trapped inside the prostate over 30 or 40 years, might trigger prostate cancer.

Urologist Ronald Wheeler speculates that chronic prostatitis may lead to prostate cancer in the same way that Barret's esophagitis may result in the development of esophageal cancer.[31] Basically, chronic inflammation leads to cancer. In an article about slow-acting bacteria and disease, Martin J. Blaser, MD, writes:

> "Consider that slow-acting bacteria, *H. Pylori*, cause a chronic inflammatory process, peptic ulcer disease, that was heretofore considered metabolic. And also keep in mind that this infection greatly enhances the risk of neoplasms developing, such as adenocarcinomas and lymphomas. It seems reasonable, then, to suggest that persistent microbes may be involved in the etiology of other chronic inflammatory diseases of unknown origin, such as . . . carcinomas of the . . . prostate."[32]

It's frightening that chronic inflammation is known to cause many kinds of cancer. Especially, since in these days of prostate specific antigen (PSA) testing, over 50 percent of men biopsied for prostate cancer will have the prostatitis lesion present whether they have cancer or not.[33] Since no one knows what causes most prostatitis (that is, inflammation of the prostate) no one knows if prostatitis causes cancer.

There is clearly an association between chronic inflammation and cancer, and the fact is, that men more often than not have inflammatory lesions in their prostate glands. These lesions occur early in life and an epidemic of prostate cancer and BPH occurs decades later. These

---

[31] Ronald E. Wheeler, MD: A Case Report of an Untold Epidemic – Prostatitis 1999. Unpublished article. Referenced with signed, written permission.
[32] Blaser MJ: The Bacteria behind Ulcers. *Scientific American*. February 1996, p. 107. Quoted with signed, written permission.
[33]Gottesman SS, Gottesman JE, Tickman, RJ: Abstract presented by JE Gottesman at 1996 American Urological Association Annual Meeting. (Similar findings also reported by pathologist John McNeal, Stanford.)

correlations cannot be dismissed without proof that they are not truly related.

Cancer-Causing Virus

Oncogenes, or cancer promoting genes, were discovered in the 1970's. When oncogenes are turned on, cells turn cancerous. Harold Varmus, a former director of the National Institutes of Health, won the Nobel Prize for finding that the Rous sarcoma virus could turn a muscle cell in a Petri dish into cancer overnight. He proved the existence of a cancer causing infection. David Baltimore, another Nobel Prize winner, theorized that retroviruses could insert themselves into DNA and be passed from parent to child through the sperm or the egg—thus making an infectious cancer appear to be inherited. In fact, the scientific world now theorizes that there are slow viruses and slow bacteria that can cause cancer decades down the road.

Prostatitis and the PSA Test

Many men, especially older men, who have prostate cancer will first become aware of it when they come down with prostatitis. The problem is that prostatitis throws off the value of the PSA test as a screen for prostate cancer. Remember that prostatitis may be the number one cause of an elevated PSA level. Solving prostatitis should make the PSA test for cancer far more sensitive, thus preventing needless biopsies.

There has been an explosion of prostate cancer biopsies and surgery because of the invention of the PSA test. Many people believe much of this poking and cutting is unnecessary, and much of the confusion is due to prostatitis.

It amazes me how many researchers will say that they feel there has to be a connection between prostatitis and prostate cancer. Yet, few if any, seem to be researching this possibility.

We already know that there are many associations between microbes and cancer. We need to solve prostatitis and we need to discover what microbes are doing inside of the prostate. In theory, even "normal flora" trapped in an obstructed prostatic sac may cause cancer over decades of time; even Staphylococcus and Streptococcus, which are normally found all over the body, if trapped inside the prostate, could be the bacteria that generate toxins and waste that lead to cancer.

Microbes may be co-factors in causing cancer. One study has shown that cancer in the presence of microbes is more virulent. In one study, germs were added to cancers in mice and the time to death from the cancer was shortened. The authors suggest that microbes make cancer more aggressive.[34] Therefore, we must learn if microbes don't directly cause cancer, do they instead make cancer more aggressive?

The Bottom Line

The bottom line is that if you have any kind of prostate trouble, including a PSA test, you need to be tested for prostatitis. If you ever have a biopsy of the prostate, be sure that they look for, and report prostatitis, if it is present.

Microbes Associated with Cancer

Here's a list of microbes and the cancers that have been associated with them:

---

[34] Shevliagin VIa, Borodina NP, Snegireva AE, Shaposhnikova GM: [Infectious risk factors in the development of malignant neoplasms]. [Article in Russian]. *Zh Mikrobiol Epidemiol Immunobiol.* 1995 Jul;4:40-42.

- Human papilloma virus has been associated with prostate cancer in some studies.
- Shistosomiasis, a parasitic disease, has been linked to prostate cancer in men in certain areas of the world
- Human papilloma virus types 16 and 18 are thought to cause cervical cancer
- Human papilloma virus types 5 and 7 are thought to cause a rare type of skin cancer (epidermodysplasia verruciformis)
- The bacteria, *Helicobacter pylori*, has been strongly associated with stomach cancer
- Epstein-Barr virus is thought to cause both African Burkitt's lymphoma and nasophayngeal carcinoma, and is associated with breast cancer.
- Human T-cell Lymphotropic virus type 1 (HTLV-1) is thought to cause adult T-cell leukemia
- Human T-cell Lymphotrophic virus type 3 (HTLV-III) is thought to cause hairy cell leukemia
- Bilharzia, a parasite, is thought to cause stomach and bladder cancer
- Feline Leukemia virus is though to cause Feline Leukemia (leukemia in cats)
- In mice, the retrovirus, mouse mammary tumor virus, is transmitted from mother to offspring. It acts like and inherited cancer, triggering breast cancer in the daughters when stimulated by the hormones of lactation
- Salmonella bacteria have been correlated with cancer of the gallbladder
- *Streptococcus bovis* has been associated with colon cancer
- Human immunodeficiency virus-type 1 (HIV) is strongly associated with Kaposi's sarcoma
- Hepatitis B is associated with hepatocellular carcinoma.
- Some researchers support an association between human papilloma virus and penile cancer
- Hepatititis C may, like Hepatitis B, also be associated with liver cancer

- Bovine papilloma virus is a suspect in equine sarcoidosis (cancer in horses)
- Avian sarcoma virus is thought to cause cancer in chickens
- The roundworm *Trichuris vulpis* is associated with esophageal cancer in dogs.

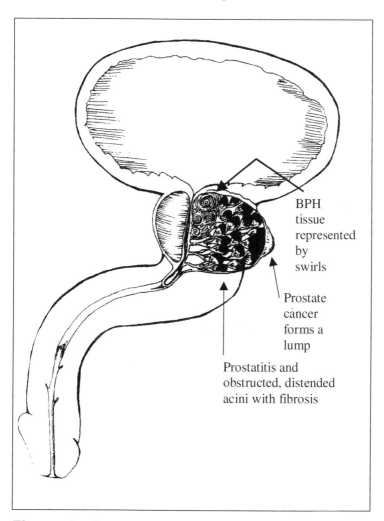

BPH tissue represented by swirls

Prostate cancer forms a lump

Prostatitis and obstructed, distended acini with fibrosis

Figure 8. As men get older, their prostates suffer from prostatitis and obstructed acini, BPH, and prostate cancer.

Staging Prostate Cancer

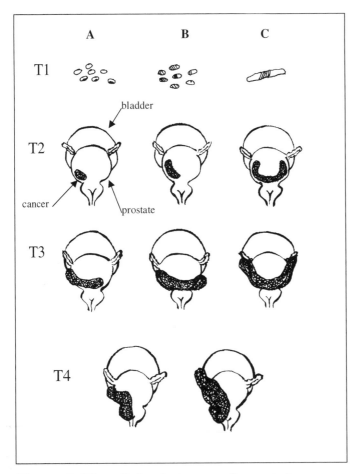

Figure 9. The clinical stages of prostate cancer are T1, T2, T3, and T4. Stage T1 is found only during a transurethral resection of the prostate (TURP), or from a needle biopsy of the prostate. Stages T2, T3 and T4 can be felt during the digital rectal examination (DRE). (Artist: Jun Macam)

The TNM Staging System

While "clinical staging" sounds complicated, it's actually a very simple concept. Your doctor stages prostate cancer by feeling for it with his gloved finger in your rectum. Your doctor palpates the cancer, determines how big it is, and whether it has escaped the prostate.

There are two types of prostate cancer, localized and escaped-from-the-prostate. Localized prostate cancer is contained inside the prostate, while more serious prostate cancer has spread, or escaped, beyond the prostate. More specifically, doctors categorize prostate cancer into four stages.

The clinical stages of prostate cancer are T1, T2, T3, and T4. T1 means that the doctor cannot feel any prostate cancer with his finger. Instead, T1 cancers are found by three methods, and are divided into substages a, b, and c. T1(a) prostate cancer is found by accident in men who have undergone a transurethral resection of the prostate—the "rotor-rooter" operation—for benign prostatic hyperplasia (BPH). To be called T1(a), prostate cancer must be found in less than 5 percent of the tissue removed during the TURP.

T1(b) means that more than 5 percent of the tissue taken out during a TURP has cancer inside it. About 10 percent of men who undergo a TURP for BPH are diagnosed with prostate cancer. It is possible that a TURP will actually remove all the prostate cancer inside a man, especially in stage T1a.

T1(c) prostate cancer, which also cannot be felt by the doctor's finger, is found because of an elevated PSA level, which prompts the doctor to do a biopsy. If the biopsy is positive for cancer, stage T1(c) exists. Stage T1(c) is diagnosed with increasing frequency as more and more men undergo biopsies for elevated PSA levels. In fact, it has become the most common stage of prostate cancer at diagnosis.

T2 cancers are also divided into a, b, and c. These cancers can all be felt as lumps on the prostate during the digital rectal exam. T2(a) prostate cancer is felt on one side of the prostate only, and involves less than 50 percent of that side.

T2(b) prostate cancer can be felt on only one side of the prostate, but involves more than 50 percent of that side. T2(c) prostate cancer is felt on both sides of the prostate. Stage T2 cancers have not yet escaped the prostate gland itself—at least as far as your doctor can tell with his or her finger.

Today, over 70 percent of men who are diagnosed with prostate cancer have clinically localized disease—the cancer has not yet escaped their prostate—as far as doctors can tell from their examinations and follow-up tests. This means that the majority of all men diagnosed with prostate cancer are at stage T1 or T2—they have localized prostate cancer contained within the prostate.

T3 prostate cancers have already escaped the prostate and are growing on the outside of it. T3(a) prostate cancer has escaped from one side of the prostate. T3(b) prostate cancer has escaped from both sides of the prostate. T3(c) prostate cancer has escaped both sides of the prostate and has invaded one or both seminal vesicles.

Stage T4 prostate cancer is the most severe. There are two kinds, a and b. T4(a) cancer has escaped the prostate and has invaded the bladder neck, rectum, or external urinary sphincter. T4(b) prostate cancer has invaded structures below the prostate (such as the levator muscle or pelvic floor).

One theory is that all prostate cancer starts out as stage T1, and over time, if a man doesn't die of something else over the years, it will turn into metastatic stage T4 prostate cancer. According to this common theory prostate cancer becomes worse over time like this:

T1 -------→T2 -------→T3 -------→T4

Rounding out this system, which is known as the TNM staging system, prostate cancer is said to be "N positive" if the lymph *nodes* are positive for cancer, and "M positive" if the cancer has *metastasized* to the bones. Thus a man is T4(b), N+, M+ if he has palpable prostate cancer spreading into the pelvic floor, positive lymph nodes, and metastases to his bones.

Unfortunately, the clinical staging of prostate cancer is not an exact science. It depends upon whether, and to what degree, the doctor's finger is perceptive. Two different doctors might stage the same man differently.

The American Joint Committee on Cancer (AJCC) and the International Union Against Cancer devised the TNM staging system.

The ABCD Staging System

There is an older and less sophisticated staging system for prostate cancer. It uses the letters ABCD, where A, B, C, and D loosely correspond to the T1, T2, T3, and T4 used above. Stage A means that prostate cancer is present but cannot be felt on digital rectal exam. Stage B is prostate cancer that can be felt during the digital rectal exam but is confined to the prostate. Stage C prostate cancers have spread outside the prostate to adjacent local tissues. Stage D prostate cancer has metastasized to the lymph nodes, the bones, or other parts of the body such as the liver or lungs.

The ABCD system is also called the "Jewett system" and is not considered as precise as the TNM system described above. Urologists tend to use it, while other doctors use the TNM system.

Gleason Grades and Scores

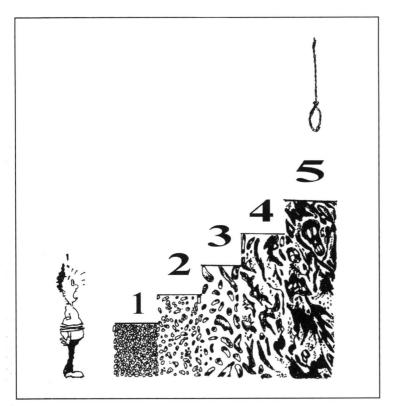

Figure 10. When the pathologist looks at your prostate cancer under the microscope, he or she gives it a grade from 1 to 5. Grade 1 looks pretty normal, but as the grade worsens to 5, prostate cancer becomes bizarrely shaped. Gleason grade 5 represents the most serious form of prostate cancer. (Artist: Jun Macam)

Introduction

Dr. Donald Gleason, a brilliant pathologist, invented the grading system for prostate cancer that now bears his name. It wasn't easy for him to come up with his 1 to 5 system of grading prostate cancer. He told me that he worried about whether or not to even call low-grade tumors cancer. He made the point that some low-grade prostate tumors are so slow-growing that they are seldom a source of bother to men; only a fraction of them ever cause symptoms and even fewer cause death.[35]

Prostate cancer is graded under the microscope, and the pathologist's eye becomes all-important when it comes to assigning a Gleason grade.

Gleason grades go from 1 to 5, with 5 being the worst. Grade 1 represents well-differentiated prostate cancer, which means that it still looks pretty similar to what normal, non-cancerous prostate tissue looks like. Gleason grade 1 retains nice, round cells that form sacs (acini), which secrete prostatic fluid. (Remember that prostatic fluid makes up part of the semen.)

But as prostate cancer progresses from Gleason grade 1 to Gleason grade 5 it becomes bizarrely shaped. The nucleus of each cancerous cell starts to fill the entire cell, making the cells appear dark and black under the microscope. The cells no longer communicate properly or form nice round acini. Gleason grade 5 prostate cancer cells look different than normal tissue found anywhere else in the body. Gleason grade 5 is shapeless and formless, a state that doctors call undifferentiated.

When the pathologist looks at a prostate cancer sample under the microscope he actually sees several Gleason grades inside the sample. Prostate cancer tumors are rarely just one grade. To deal with multiple grades of cancer inside one tumor, the Gleason *score* is used. The

---

[35] Gleason, Donald: Telephone conversation with the author. August 16, 1998, with signed, written permission.

Gleason score equals the most common Gleason grade *plus* the second most common Gleason grade.

So first, the pathologist determines the most common Gleason *grade* that he sees on your slide. Next, he verifies the second most common Gleason grade. These two grades are added together to give the Gleason *score*. For example, if you have mostly Gleason grade 3 prostate cancer, and have Gleason grade 2 as the next most common grade, you have a Gleason score of 5, because (3 + 2) = 5. *Gleason grades* go from 1 to 5, while *Gleason scores* range from 2 to 10.

Gleason scores roughly correlate with the aggressiveness of prostate cancer. In general, the higher the Gleason score the more likely the prostate cancer is to grow, spread, and kill a man. This is, however, a generalization. Physicians wish that the Gleason score could predict exactly what prostate cancer will do. Unfortunately, the Gleason score can't predict exactly what prostate cancer will do, but it does give us trends.

Part of the problem is that we have no way of determining how long a cancer has been present before being discovered. Autopsy studies indicate that some low-grade tumors are probably present for ten, twenty, or thirty years before diagnosis. What's involved is a race between tumor growth and dying from other causes. But we don't know the day the prostate cancer first appeared, so it's like watching a race after it has started. Somewhere in the middle, we tune in to the race, but we don't know when the finish line will appear either. Yet, the race is on between tumor growth and the end of a man's life by other causes.

Gleason in medical studies

When medical studies are done, things can become confusing. In studies, Gleason scores are often lumped together to describe low, medium, or high-grade cancer. Low-grade consists of Gleason scores 2, 3, and 4. Medium-grade prostate cancer is represented by Gleason scores 5, 6, and 7. High-grade prostate cancer means Gleason scores of 8, 9, and 10.

All this can be confusing because studies don't always spell out these distinctions. And watch out for a Gleason score of 7. It may not be appropriate to lump it with Gleason scores of 5 and 6, as it sometimes acts more like high-grade prostate cancer than medium-grade cancer. Gleason grade 7 may behave in either slow-growing fashion or aggressive fashion, and there is no way to tell which way it will behave in a particular man.

Low-grade prostate cancer is slow-growing and the overwhelming majority of men never die from it. Medium-grade prostate cancer is the most common prostate cancer. High-grade prostate cancer is relatively rare but has the worst prognosis. High-grade prostate cancer carries the greatest risk of being metastatic at the time of diagnosis. For instance, one study found that high-grade prostate cancer is associated with a 75 to 100 percent chance that the cancer has spread to the lymph nodes.[36]

Differences Between Differentiated and Undifferentiated Prostate Cancer

Some studies like to talk in terms of differentiation instead of low-grade, medium-grade, and high-grade cancer. Gleason scores of 2, 3, and 4 are considered "well-differentiated." Gleason scores of 5, 6, and 7 are considered "moderately differentiated," and Gleason scores of 8, 9, and 10 are considered "undifferentiated." I prefer using the terms "low-grade," "medium-grade," and "high-grade" prostate cancer, and I use those terms throughout this book.

---

[36] Plawker MW, Fleisher JM, Vapnek EM, and Macchia RJ: Current trends in prostate cancer diagnosis and staging among United States urologists. *Journal of Urology*, November 1997;158:1853-1858.

One Study in JAMA

One study in the *Journal of the American Medical Association* estimated the probability of dying from localized prostate cancer, or other competing causes of death, depending upon the Gleason scores. The study covered a 15-year period.[37] The results are summarized in the table below:

Gleason Scores	Risk of dying from prostate cancer over 15 years instead of something else
2 to 4	4 to 7 percent
5	6 to 11 percent
6	18 to 30 percent
7	42 to 70 percent
8 to 10	60 to 87 percent

Note in the table above that the Gleason score of 7 is quite different in terms of the risk of dying than a Gleason score of 5 or 6. Again, this is noteworthy because many studies group Gleason scores 5, 6, and 7 together, calling them all medium-grade prostate cancer.

One way to look at the table above is "Oh my God, I'm going to die." Another way to look at it is how often treatment is not needed. Most men in the study had prostate cancer with Gleason scores ranging from 2 to 6. Their risk of dying from prostate cancer only ranges from 4 to 30 percent. This is the conundrum of prostate cancer— the majority of men with it do not need treatment to survive it.

---

[37] Albertsen PC, Hanley JA, Gleason DF, and Barry MJ: Competing Risk Analysis of Men Aged 55 to 74 Years at Diagnosis Managed Conservatively for Clinically Localized Prostate Cancer. JAMA 1998;280(11):975-980. Adapted table 3. Copyright 1998, American Medical Association. Quoted with signed, written permission.

Not Perfect

The Gleason score is helpful, but doesn't tell us all we want to know. There is no perfect way to tell slow-growing prostate cancer from fast-growing prostate cancer. Things are never simple with prostate cancer. A patient can have a high-Gleason-score cancer that never kills him; while infrequently, another man can have a low-Gleason-score cancer that does kill him. What is true is that as the Gleason score goes up, a man is more likely to succumb to prostate cancer over the years than to die of some other cause.

One warning about Gleason scoring is that it is not an exact science. It's a process of recognizing patterns under the microscope. You can show the same prostate cancer slide to two different pathologists who may well arrive at different Gleason scores. Several oncologists have advised me that it is important for the patient to know that Gleason grading is somewhat subjective. You may want a second opinion about your Gleason score from the most qualified prostate cancer pathologist available before considering any treatment.

DNA Ploidy Status

Besides using the microscope to ascertain Gleason grades and scores, there is another approach that can be helpful in telling how likely prostate cancer is to metastasize. It's the DNA Ploidy test, in which cells from the prostate biopsy are stained so that they will fluoresce under a black light. This causes their chromosomes to light up. The closer the chromosomes are to those in normal prostate tissue the better. As the chromosomes become more numerous, less structured, and more bizarre, the cancer's aggressiveness increases.

"Diploid" is the term for a normal result. We humans have two sets of chromosomes; thus the term "diploid" designates normal for us. Tetraploid means "four ploidy," or double the two sets of chromosomes normally found in each cell. Having double the number of chromosomes means that the cancer is getting worse. Tumors that are most aggressive and most likely to metastasize are referred to as "aneuploid." Aneuploid means not normal (an = not, and euploid = normal). Aneuploid tumors have more than double the normal number of chromosomes—their chromosomes may fill up almost all of each cell.

One study from the Mayo Clinic pointed out how significant aneuploidy is as a bad prognostic sign.[38] It involved 261 men with clinically localized prostate cancer who underwent surgery. Examination of the removed prostates confirmed that the prostate cancer was contained within the prostate. Ten men in the study had aneuploid tumors and all 10 developed progression of their cancer despite surgery. The lesson is that a disproportionate number of men with aneuploidy have progression of their prostate cancer. I have tabulated the results of this important study below. Note that overall, 20 percent of these men with localized prostate cancer had a recurrence of their cancer. Therefore, the surgery, the radical prostatectomy, failed in 20 percent of men with localized prostate cancer—the 20 percent that really needed curative treatment.

Men with localized prostate cancer who underwent radical prostatectomy	Number of men who had a recurrence of their prostate cancer	Percentage of men who had a recurrence of their prostate cancer
261 men total	53	20 percent
177 diploid tumors	27	15 percent
74 tetraploid tumors	16	22 percent
10 aneuploid tumors	10	100 percent

[38] Montgomery BT, Ofer N, Blute ML, Farrow GM, Myers RP, Zinke H, Therneau TM, Lieber MM: Stage B Protate Adenocarcinoma. *Archives of Surgery.* 1990;125:327-331.

From the table, you can see that as the ploidy status worsens, prostate cancer becomes more likely to spread. There is also a relationship between Gleason scores and ploidy status. As the Gleason scores go up, there is a greater likelihood of finding tetraploid or aneuploid tumors. Only patients with high Gleason scores (6 to 10) had aneuploidy.

If ploidy status is so helpful in predicting what prostate cancer will do, why don't doctors do it all the time? In the past, the problem was that it took a lot of tissue to do ploidy analysis. The doctors in the Mayo Clinic study above needed 10,000 cells to do their ploidy tests. Currently, most prostate cancer patients undergo needle biopsies of their prostates to diagnose prostate cancer, which may only provide 100 cells.

However, the Mayo Clinic has developed a new method of doing ploidy analysis that enables them to do it on needle biopsies. The Mayo Clinic is currently doing studies to see if the new technique of ploidy analysis proves to be helpful for men who are getting biopsies for prostate cancer. It may be that ploidy analysis will turn out to be very useful. In fact, a couple of commercial laboratories have started offering both Gleason scoring and ploidy analysis on needle biopsy specimens.

If you undergo a biopsy, try to get both a Gleason score and ploidy analysis. Be sure to talk to your doctor about their availability before you undergo the biopsy procedure.

Your Prostate Specific Antigen (PSA) Level

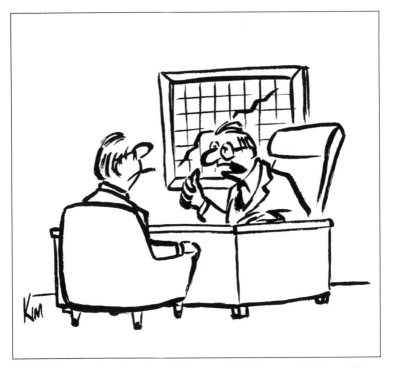

Figure 11. Urologist: "Your PSA Level? No. Those are my profits since the PSA test started finding prostate cancer in everybody." (Artist: Mike Kim).

Introduction

In 1986 the Food and Drug Administration approved the first PSA (prostate specific antigen) test for prostate cancer, which revolutionized prostate cancer detection. Today, over 70 percent of all prostate cancers are discovered by the PSA test.

Someone draws a tube of blood from your arm, it's processed in the laboratory, and within a day or two, you know what your PSA level is.

When the PSA test was first introduced, men were advised that a normal level was between 0 to 4.0 nanograms per milliliter (a nanogram is a billionth of a gram). Anything higher than 4.0 was considered suspicious for prostate cancer. Over time, however, the 4.0 ng/ml cutoff has proved less than accurate. What should be called "normal" is constantly being reevaluated. In addition, the PSA test is being used in new and novel ways.

The lesson is that the "0 to 4" ngs/ml range is now considered generally inaccurate, especially for different age groups of men, and for men of different ethnic backgrounds.

The Normal PSA Level

When a PSA level up to 4 is called normal, some prostate cancers will be missed. The American Cancer Society emphasizes that a "normal" PSA of less than 4.0 ng/ml doesn't rule out prostate cancer in all patients. The Society points out that about 25 percent of men with prostate cancer will have a PSA of less than 4.0 at diagnosis.[39]

More recently, one group studied 2,950 men (age range 62 – 91 years) for seven years, all of whom never had a PSA level of more than 4.0 ng per milliliter. After undergoing biopsy, prostate cancer was diagnosed in 15 percent of the men. Within the group, the higher the PSA level within the range of 0 – 4, the more likely prostate cancer was to be diagnosed. Surprisingly, 15 percent of the 15 percent of men in whom prostate cancer was diagnosed had high-grade prostate cancer.[40]

---

[39] American Cancer Society Prostate Screening Guidelines. 1997.
[40] Thompson IM, Pauler DK, Goodman PJ, Tangen CM, Lucia MS, Parnes HL, Minasian LM, Ford LG, Lippman SM, Crawford ED, Crowley JJ, Coltman CA Jr.: Prevalence of prostate cancer among men with a prostate-specific antigen level

The other side of the coin, however, is that even when elevated above 4.0, the PSA test is not completely accurate. Some studies show that only about 25 percent of men with a PSA over 4.0 and as high as 10.0 actually have prostate cancer discovered on biopsy. The rest exhibit elevated PSA levels due to prostatitis, benign prostatic hyperplasia (BPH), or laboratory error. This means that using the 4.0 cutoff results in a lot of unnecessary biopsies – unnecessary needles thrust into your body through your rectum! In general, the higher the PSA the more likely that the elevation is due to prostate cancer.

What is Normal?

Doctors are reconsidering what should be called a normal PSA level. Dr. Ferndand Labrie, an endocrinologist and leading prostate cancer expert, believes that a PSA level over 3.0 should be considered the cutoff for prostate cancer detection. Dr. Duke Bahn, a radiologist and cryosurgeon, believes that 2.0 should be the upper limit of normal. And urologist Ronald Wheeler believes that 1.0 should be the cutoff for normal, because a PSA level above 1.0 almost always means that prostatitis, benign prostatic hyperplasia (BPH), or prostate cancer are present.

PSA Greater than 1 is Abnormal

I agree with Dr. Wheeler that a PSA level above 1.0 is abnormal, and that prostatitis and BPH should not be ignored. If you are found to have a PSA greater than 1.0 be sure to be tested for prostatitis and BPH, in addition to being followed for prostate cancer. Prostatitis and BPH should be diagnosed and treated as described in my previous book, *The Prostatitis Syndromes*, or in my upcoming book, *Prostatitis and BPH*. I believe urologists'

< or =4.0 ng per milliliter. *New England Journal of Medicine.* 2004 May 27;350(22):2239-46.

failure to diagnose prostatitis and BPH is the single greatest problem with the PSA test.

The Leaky Prostate

One patient described having an elevated PSA as having a "leaky prostate." I think that's a good way to look at it. The more diseased your prostate, the more likely your prostate is to be swollen and to be leaking its PSA into your bloodstream, and the more likely you are to be suffering from prostatitis, BPH, or prostate cancer. And if you have prostate cancer, perhaps the leakier your prostate is, the more likely the cancer is to spread.

Prostatitis is a Big Problem

Many sources consider prostatitis the number one cause of a falsely elevated PSA level. A growing number of physicians first treat men with elevated PSA levels for prostatitis, and then, only if the PSA is still elevated after such treatment, proceed to biopsy. Treating prostatitis will allow many biopsies to be avoided. Unfortunately, it's common for many doctors to focus on prostate cancer alone.

Dr. Wheeler says:

> "A PSA greater than 1 is abnormal. If it's over 1, the man is suffering from prostatitis, BPH, or prostate cancer, with prostatitis being the most likely."[41]

Prostatitis and BPH interfere greatly with the accuracy of the PSA test for prostate cancer. One study found that if 100 men over the age of fifty were tested, ten would have an elevated PSA. Of these ten, only three will actually have

---

[41] Ronald E. Wheeler, MD: Telephone conversation with the author April 22, 1999. Quoted with signed, written permission.

prostate cancer.[42] Seven out of 10 men thus receive unnecessary biopsies according to this source.

We need to make a concerted effort to keep men's prostates small and PSA levels below 1.0 throughout life instead of watching the PSA slowly rise with age. My companion book to this one suggests ways in which this might be done. It's wrong to be cavalier about letting the prostate deteriorate, as evidenced by rising PSA levels with age, while standing by and doing nothing. Why allow PSA levels as high as 4.0 to be called normal, when anything over 1.0 probably indicates disease? Clearly doctors can step in much earlier to treat prostatitis and BPH, and possibly prevent prostate cancer.

Age-Adjusted PSA

Because men accumulate prostatitis and BPH in their prostates as they age, sometimes age-adjusted PSA levels are used for prostate cancer detection. For example, more than one source suggests that when it comes to considering a biopsy, men less than 50 years of age should have PSAs under 2.5, while men 70 to 79 can have PSA levels approaching 6.5 without cancer, because of all the BPH and prostatitis inside them.

Repeat the Test

If you have your PSA level tested and it is elevated, the first thing a conscientious physician usually does is repeat the test. One deficiency of the PSA test is that its results can fluctuate widely between measurements done a short time apart. The authors of one study suggest that

---

[42] Institute For Clinical Evaluative Sciences in Ontario. PSA Screening-Physician information.1997. Available at http://www.ices.on.ca/docs/fb1231a.htm.

before a biopsy is undertaken, two, or even three, PSA tests might be warranted.[43]

Reproducibility

If you are being screened for prostate cancer or for a recurrence of prostate cancer after treatment, you want to be certain that fluctuations in the results aren't due to the test itself. Otherwise, variations in the results could lead you to believe erroneously that you have cancer, or a recurrence of cancer. You and your physician must discuss the reliability of the PSA tests available to you. You should attempt to have the same laboratory run your PSA test each time, and attempt to go into each test under the same conditions.

False PSA Elevations

Several things may elevate the PSA level: prostatitis, BPH, prostate cancer, laboratory error, the drug allopurinol (which is used for gout), digital rectal examination, prostatic massage, prostatic ultrasound, and biopsy of the prostate.

There is conflicting information about whether the digital rectal exam elevates the PSA. WARNING: Be wary of urologists who do a digital rectal exam, or prostatic massage, before drawing your blood for a PSA test. A sinister or incompetent doctor could potentially drive your PSA level up by such a maneuver, especially one who is looking to do more biopsies and surgeries.

There is conflicting data about whether the insertion of a urinary catheter might elevate the PSA. Studies also conflict over whether sexual activity raises the PSA level.

Some sources suggest not ejaculating seventy-two hours prior to being tested. Others sources, realizing that

---

[43] Roehrborn CG, Pikens GJ, and Carmody III T: Variability of repeated serum prostate-specific antigen (PSA) measurements within less than 90 days in a well-defined patient population. UROLOGY. 1996;47(1):59-66.

abstinence is difficult for many men, suggest making sure that prior sexual activity, or lack thereof, is the same before each PSA test is performed.

On the other hand, the PSA level is lowered by Proscar (finasteride), a commonly prescribed BPH medication. Therefore, many doctors suggest a baseline PSA level should be obtained before starting Proscar.

The Rise of the PSA

Several things can be done to enhance the accuracy of the PSA test. For example, doctors are realizing that not only is the PSA level important, but that the rise of the PSA within the normal range should be looked at carefully. If you have a PSA level of 1.5 and it goes to 3.0, even though both are still "normal" levels, you should be concerned.

Gleason Grade Three is Unique

Keep in mind that Gleason grade 3 tumors (remember, grades go from 1 to 5) are thought to be the biggest producers of PSA.

Some high-grade tumors don't produce a lot of PSA. Some of these undifferentiated tumors have "forgotten how" or lost the ability to produce PSA. This further confuses doctors and patients. Which is worse, grade 5 prostate cancer with a low PSA, or grade 3 prostate cancer with a high PSA?

PSA Velocity

How quickly your PSA test goes up over time can help you tell whether or not you have prostate cancer. This is called PSA velocity. Ideally, PSA velocity should be based on at least two different PSA determinations, twelve months apart. However, a projection can be made from PSA tests done closer together. Blood collected for each PSA test should be drawn under similar circumstances and tested by the same laboratory. A rise equivalent to 0.75 per year is considered worrisome. Some experts are currently recommending a prostate biopsy when such a rise occurs, thinking that such a rapid rise in PSA points towards prostate cancer. Importantly, according to one study by Dr. Anthony D'Amico, a PSA velocity of 2.0 nanograms per milliliter per year or greater, is a strong predictive factor for eventual death from prostate cancer.[44]

PSA Doubling Time

Another variation in PSA testing is the PSA doubling time. Remember that prostate cancer grows exponentially. That is, every cell divides, so you go from 2 cells to 4, 8, 16, 32, 64 and so on. With the tumor frequently doubling in size, the amount of PSA produced may double also, so calculating PSA doubling time may help us. Scientists are attempting to work out exactly what values for PSA doubling time are abnormal.

PSA Density

To calculate PSA density, the PSA level is divided by the size of the prostate as measured by transrectal ultrasound or magnetic resonance imaging. PSA density is another tool being developed for trying to establish whether an elevated PSA is due to prostate cancer or to a noncancerous condition. Current thinking is that the PSA density will help tell BPH from prostate cancer, especially in men with PSA elevations from 4 to 10. Men in this range who have an elevated PSA density are thought to be at an increased risk for prostate cancer. Patients who have a PSA from 4 to 10, who have a low PSA density, are thought to be more likely to have BPH. The problem with PSA density is

---

[44] Anthony V. D'Amico, MD, PhD, Ming-Hui Chen, PhD, Kimberly A. Roehl, MPH, and William J. Catalona, MD: *The New England Journal of Medicine*, July 8, 2004; vol 351: pp 125-135.

that our measurements of prostate volume with ultrasound or MRI are not as accurate as we would like, which throws off the numbers. The second thing is that PSA density can't account for prostatitis.

Race Matters when Testing the PSA

PSA levels vary between the races. It's important not to use the standard for one ethnic group as the standard for another ethnic group. Urologist Joseph Oesterling has suggested the following guidelines where both age and ethnic origin are taken into account. Ages are listed in the left column, while normal PSA ranges for Blacks, Caucasians, and Japanese men are listed to the right.

Age-Specific Reference Ranges for Serum PSA[45]

Age Range (Years)	Reference Range (ng/ml)		
	Blacks	Caucasians	Japanese
40-49	0.0-2.0	0.0-2.5	0.0-2.0
50-59	0.0-4.0	0.0-3.5	0.0-3.0
60-69	0.0-4.5	0.0-4.5	0.0-4.0
70-79	0.0-5.5	0.0-6.5	0.0-5.0

Free PSA

Free PSA (also called PSA II) is thought to be an important new test that can help tell if elevations in PSA are due to prostate cancer, BPH, or prostatitis. Remember that most men old enough to be worried about prostate cancer already have BPH and prostatitis.

---

[45] Oesterling, Joseph. Prostate Specific Antigen: Making an Excellent Tumor Marker Even Better. Mediconsult.com limited. Available at: http://mediconsult.com/associations/ustoo/back_issues/Vol1_No5/article03.html. Reproduced with signed, written permission.

Free PSA is a good thing! PSA produced by cancer cells is usually attached to a protein when it is in the bloodstream. Protein-bound PSA is associated with prostate cancer. Free PSA, on the other hand, suggests that you are cancer free. The more free PSA, or the higher the ratio of free to bound PSA, the less likely that an elevated PSA is due to prostate cancer. Scientists are still trying to calculate the appropriate ratio. Some think the free PSA should be one-fifth or one-fourth of total PSA, or higher. One study found that the free/total PSA ratio was an improvement over PSA alone, or PSA density, in telling prostate cancer from BPH.[46]

In an interesting variation, some researchers are looking at the complexed PSA instead of the free PSA component. One study found that if a cutoff for complexed-to-total PSA of 0.80 is used, the test is more sensitive than looking at free PSA ratios.[47]

Partin Tables

Urologist Alan Partin, who invented the "Partin Tables" for predicting organ confinement in prostate cancer, notes that men with PSAs between 4 and 10 have less than a 50 percent chance of having a positive biopsy for cancer. In other words, a lot of men in this group get needless biopsies. Partin suggests that in men with PSAs between 4 and 10 the risk of prostate cancer is less than 10 percent if the free PSA ratio is greater than 25 percent. If the free PSA ratio is less than 10 percent, the risk for prostate cancer is

---

[46] Akdas A, Cevik I, Tarcan T, Turkeri L, Dalaman G, and Emerk K: The role of free prostate-specific antigen in the diagnosis of prostate cancer. *British Journal of Urology*, 1997;79:920-923.

[47] España F, Royo M, Martínez M, Enguídanos MJ, Vera CD, Estellés A, Aznar J, Jiménez-Cruz JF, and Heeb MJ: Free and Complexed Prostate Specific Antigen in the Differentiation of Benign Prostatic Hyperplasia and Prostate Cancer: Studies in Serum and Plasma Samples. *The Journal of Urology*. 1998;160:2081-1998.

thought to be greater than 80 percent.[48] It is hoped that information of this kind will someday reduce the large number of unnecessary prostate biopsies. (The percentage of free PSA is the result of dividing the free PSA result by the total PSA level and multiplying by 100.)

DNA based PSA Test

Probably the most sensitive PSA test of all is one that tests for the DNA of cells that produce PSA. The test has a difficult name, RT-PCR-PSA, which stands for reverse transcriptase—polymerase chain reaction—prostate specific antigen.

Normally, men shouldn't have PSA-secreting cells floating around in their bloodstream. If this test is positive, prostate cancer has probably already escaped the prostate and has metastasized somewhere. RT-PCR-PSA assays are thought to be so sensitive that they can pick up one prostate cancer cell out of one million blood cells.[49] Studies are already being published suggesting that it's a better measure for determining whether or not a cancer is locally confined than regular PSA, Gleason grade, the digital rectal exam, or imaging of the prostate.[50]

Although the RT-PCR-PSA test is an exciting new development, further study is needed before it's adopted as invariably valid. The problem with the test is that false positives and false negatives can occur and mislead one into thinking cancer has spread when it hasn't, or that the

---

[48] Partin AW, and Carter HB: The use of prostate-specific antigen and free/total prostate-specific antigen in the diagnosis of localized prostate cancer. *Urologic Clinics of North America.* November 1996;23(4):531-540.

[49] Stephen B. Strum, MD, FACP, and Mark Scholz MD: Patients with Early Disease Part 1. New Approaches in Prostate Cancer 1994-1996. Internet World Wide Web. 1996.

[50] Katz AE, de Vries GM, Benson MC, Buttyan RE, O'Toole K, Rubin MA, Stifleman M, Olsson CA: The role of reverse-transcriptase polymerase chain reaction assay for prostate-specific antigen in the selection of patients for radical prostatectomy. *Urologic Clinics of North America.* November 1996;23(4):541-549.

cancer is contained in the prostate when it isn't. When it comes to prostate cancer, DNA testing is not infallible.

The ProstAsure Test

The ProstAsure blood test measures the PSA and four other substances in the blood. This information is plugged into a computer, which then predicts whether prostate cancer is present or not. The ProstAsure test uses a technique called "neural net analysis" to interpret the levels of the five substances. Reduced to its basics, neural net analysis is a way of taking many equations that are important to analyzing the odds of something occurring and having the computer calculate those odds. This is necessary because, with too many variables, it becomes too cumbersome for the human mind to grasp the equations and the odds that result from them. The ProstAsure test, approved by the FDA in March 1996, tells you which one of four categories applies to you: 1) normal, 2) BPH, 3) suspicious for BPH, or 4) prostate cancer. The ProstAsure test has the potential for saving men from unnecessary biopsies and increasing the accuracy of diagnosis. The test's flaw is that it can't account for prostatitis.

ProstAsure is thought to be more likely than the PSA test to find early prostate cancer. Its sensitivity is claimed to be between 80 to 85 percent, while that of the PSA test, even when combined with a digital rectal examination, is presently less than 50 percent. The ProstAsure test may be particularly helpful in men who have a PSA level below 4.0. Remember that about one-fourth or one-third of men with prostate cancer have PSA levels below 4.0. In such men, the ProstAsure test may be able to distinguish between BPH and prostate cancer. In the United States, the ProstAsure test evaluation must be ordered through a licensed physician.

Unfortunately, the ProstAsure test may have disappeared by the time this book is published. If so, it will be another good idea down the drain.

Sensitive PSA Tests

Regular PSA tests are fine for checking if the PSA is between zero and 4.0. However, when the PSA is employed for the purpose of following treatment instead of screening for cancer, sensitive PSA tests with low detection limits are needed. For example, once a radical prostatectomy is done the PSA level should go to zero and stay there. A sensitive test that can pick up any tiny rise in PSA above zero is needed to follow men for post-surgical return of cancer. Several PSA tests have been developed that can detect PSA levels in the .003 to .007 range, and these ultra-sensitive PSA tests are used to follow men after surgery, and sometimes after other forms of treatment.

The PSA Level May Suggest Metastatic Disease

The PSA test not only helps to screen for prostate cancer, but when cancer is present, it helps suggest whether it has spread beyond the prostate. The higher the PSA level, the more likely it is that the cancer has traveled outside of the prostate. For example, if the PSA is above 10, experts suggest the possibility that the cancer has spread outside the prostate as being anywhere from 15 percent to 50 percent.

On the other hand, for us to predict with good odds that prostate cancer is confined to the prostate there should be a PSA of less than 10. In fact, some experts will argue that a PSA of less than 7 should be present.

PSA Anxiety

After the radical prostatectomy, the PSA should be zero and stay zero with standard PSA tests. However as PSA tests have become more sensitive, even ultra-sensitive, following the PSA level can result in some anxiety. Currently, if the PSA level rises above 0.2

nanograms/millimeter after radical prostatectomy, it should cause concern. This is called biochemical failure, which may precede actual return of the cancer by several years. For radiation therapy, hormone blockade, and cryoablation, since the entire prostate is not removed or destroyed, PSA failure is often defined as three PSA rises in a row rather than any absolute level.

Conclusion

The attempts to make the PSA test better are very important. If we could somehow tell when the PSA is high because of prostatitis or BPH, versus prostate cancer, a lot of prostatic biopsies could be avoided. This is important because prostate biopsies are an ordeal for men, who risk pain and side effects when they undergo the procedure. In addition, we need to focus on the PSA test as a diagnostic, as well as screening test, for all three prostate diseases, prostatitis, BPH, and cancer, instead of only considering prostate cancer alone.

Making the PSA test better may not be easy. A recent provocative paper by Urologist Thomas Stamey and others screams: THE PROSTATE SPECIFIC ANTIGEN ERA IN THE UNITED STATES IS OVER FOR PROSTATE CANCER: WHAT HAPPENED IN THE LAST 20 YEARS? The paper, in the Journal of Urology, October 2004, says that the PSA test is no longer accurate for prostate cancer, only for BPH (benign prostatic hyperplasia).

THE LESSON: If your PSA level is over 1.0, you probably have prostatitis, BPH, or prostate cancer. The urological community has focused too much on prostate cancer in my opinion, while failing to provide satisfactory solutions for all the prostatitis and BPH that is being discovered by the PSA test.

The PSA Screening Debate

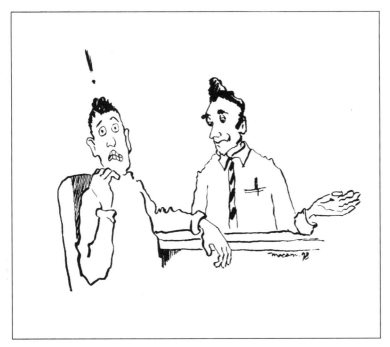

Figure 12. "Sure, I can screen you for prostate cancer with the PSA test, but then I'll have to mutilate you beyond anything you could ever comprehend if you test positive, and it will probably be all for nothing." (Artist: Jun Macam)

Introduction

Most men will be surprised to learn how controversial prostate specific antigen (PSA) testing is among academic physicians. The controversy is whether or not healthy men should be screened for prostate cancer in order to detect tumors as early as possible.

To date, most public policy people who have looked at the issue have concluded that PSA screening is of no benefit to men. This is because the controlled scientific evidence that treating prostate cancer helps men is very weak or nonexistent, while the harm done to men from treating their prostate cancer is very real. Based on hard science, it's likely that universal screening would do more harm than good because many men suffer significantly from their prostate cancer treatments.

It's important to understand; however, that the PSA test can be used either as a screening test or a diagnostic test. Men sometimes ask me, "Should I be screened for prostate cancer?"

"How old are you?" I ask, and then I follow that question with a series of others: "Do you ever wake up at night to urinate? Do you ever dribble after urination? Do you urinate more often than you used to? Has your sexual function declined? Are your erections less hard or less frequent? Is your orgasm less powerful? Is you semen lesser in quantity? Do you ever have trouble getting started urinating in a public restroom?" Most of the time, when a man asks me about the PSA test, careful questioning will reveal that he has one or more symptoms that could be related to the prostate.

I then explain that the PSA test is being used as a screening test only when it is performed on men who have no symptoms whatsoever. It's being used as a diagnostic test when it's done on men who already have symptoms.

I continue by saying, "You already have some symptoms that could be attributed to your prostate. You need to have the PSA test to help diagnose why you are having these symptoms, and in particular to sort out if they might be due to prostatitis, benign prostatic hyperplasia (BPH), or prostate cancer." In other words, often men think they are being screened for prostate cancer when in reality they need the test to help diagnose some symptom that they already have. Most men getting a PSA test are over fifty years old, and accordingly, have prostate-related symptoms.

There is really no controversy in doing the PSA test for men with symptoms. The controversy is only whether men with no symptoms should be PSA-screened for prostate cancer.

We Don't Screen Because Surgery is a Failure

If surgery absolutely worked to cure prostate cancer, today we would be screening all men for prostate cancer. But surgery has already failed two controlled studies (to be examined later), and since, despite its failure, surgery is the "gold standard" prostate cancer treatment offered by urologists, the United States Government currently sees no net benefit from PSA screening for prostate cancer.

Digital Rectal Exam

There are actually two screening tests for prostate cancer. Besides the PSA test there is the digital rectal exam (DRE). The DRE is done as part of a routine physical, costs nothing extra, and screens for both colon cancer and prostate cancer. Some men with prostate cancer never have an elevated PSA, but their cancer can be felt during the DRE. This is why the digital rectal examination should not be skipped. Done together, the PSA test and the DRE are superior to either test alone. I'm a believer in the DRE because doctors need to examine all their patients as completely as they can.

Your doctor should do the PSA test first, as the DRE could cause a rise in the PSA level.

Take Home Message

I think that men most men, middle-aged and older, should want a PSA test, and when it is found to be over 1.0, should have tests for prostatitis first and foremost, before going on to be investigated for BPH and prostate cancer.

Moe and Larry's Diagnosis of Prostate Cancer

Moe and Larry are worried about prostate cancer. Moe has an elevated PSA level of 8.0, while Larry's doctor discovered a lump on the left side of his prostate during a digital rectal exam. What happens to Moe and Larry now?

Moe's doctor calls him to come in for a digital rectal exam, which is free of any lumps. The doctor repeats Moe's PSA level and it is still 8.0, which helps to rule out laboratory error as the cause of the elevation. Moe's family physician carefully interviews him for symptoms of prostatitis. He also checks Moe's prostatic fluid several times during separate visits to completely rule out prostatitis as the cause of Moe's elevated PSA level.

Larry's doctor, because of Larry's prostate lump, tests Larry's PSA level and it's high, it's 16. A repeat level is also 16. Larry is also told that, besides the lump, his prostate is enlarged. Larry's doctor won't check for prostatitis and Larry lets it slide.

Moe and Larry now know their PSA levels and what their prostates feel like during the digital rectal exam. Moe also knows that he does not have prostatitis.

Moe and Larry need to stop and learn about prostate cancer before proceeding to biopsy. A biopsy is when a doctor sticks a needle into the prostate to get a little piece of it to look at under the microscope. A biopsy, if it samples the right area, can prove that prostate cancer is present; however, there are risks to having a biopsy. I'm going to explain them in detail a little bit later.

Once educated about prostate cancer treatments, some men will decide against undergoing a biopsy. In addition, there are some tests Moe and Larry could have that might forestall the need for a biopsy.

Moe and Larry both go for transrectal ultrasound of the prostate (TRUS). With TRUS a probe is inserted into the rectum and sound waves are used to visualize the prostate. It is sometimes possible to see a likely area for prostate cancer with ultrasound. Suspicious areas are targeted for biopsy. The original ultrasound machines were black and white. Newer, color Doppler ultrasound machines are available and may be better at detecting prostate disease.

Moe's TRUS is normal, while Larry's shows a suspicious area where his lump is and confirms that his prostate is enlarged. Both men resist the pressure to "just have a biopsy done" during their first TRUS. They want to know the results of the TRUS, and to digest those results, before allowing needles to be stuck inside their bodies. Moe and Larry are intelligent men. Like Moe and Larry, whatever you do or don't do, be wary of sitting back and letting others make all the decisions.

Moe and Larry decide to have other tests done before jumping to biopsy. They both have their free PSA measured and their PSA density calculated. They will each have their PSA redrawn in a month so that their PSA velocity can be projected. Unfortunately for Moe and Larry, their free PSA levels suggest prostate cancer. Their PSA density calculations also suggest prostate cancer.

Moe and Larry have to fight to get RT-PCR-PSA testing done. Their physician doesn't want to do it before they have biopsies. They insist. They get the difficult-to-arrange test done and no evidence of metastatic prostate cancer is found in either man.

Moe and Larry also have to be aggressive in order to get the ProstAsure test done. The ProstAsure test analyzes PSA plus four other biomarkers from the blood. A computer analyzes the significance of the biomarkers. Moe and Larry's ProstAsure tests indicate that they probably have prostate cancer and that Larry has BPH as well.

Acid Phosphatase

Men with an elevated prostatic acid phosphatase are at an increased risk for metastatic prostate cancer. Fortunately, both Moe and Larry have low levels of the enzyme.

Viagra

I advise Moe and Larry to try Viagra (sildenafil). Moe and Larry say things have slowed down sexually, but that there is no definite problem. I want Moe and Larry to know what Viagra can do for them, and to be aware of how good their sex lives can be, before any potentially harmful procedure is performed on them. In the very near future they may have to make decisions that could impact their sexual function.

Moe and Larry are both delighted to find that Viagra gives them harder, better erections. They both feel more committed to saving their sex lives after trying the medication.

Moe and Larry decide to learn more about prostate biopsies, but what they read in the newspaper, horrifies them.

Headlines

"ANGRY PATIENT VANDALIZED DOCOTORS' OFFICES" and "PROSTATE PATIENT GOES CRAZY" screamed the newspaper headlines in the spring of 2000. Sixty-five-year old John J. Murphy, a retired accountant for Western Electric Bell System, became understandably upset when urologists would not, or could not help him with his prostate problems. He shattered windows and spray-painted over urologists' names at a dozen urologists' offices. Why was Mr. Murphy so upset? Because he went for help with getting up 5 to 10 times per night to urinate and instead of helping his symptoms, they biopsied—twice no less—his prostate, and made his symptoms worse! For his act of civil disobedience, Mr. Murphy spent 3 months in jail, was given 5-years probation, and still has lawsuits pending against him.[51]

According to Mr. Murphy, not a single urologist bothered to massage his prostate and collect his prostatic fluid for analysis!

Whatever happened, and I am not saying that anything was done wrong for Mr. Murphy; the point is that urologists made him worse instead of better. For the diagnosis and treatment of prostatitis and BPH you need to see my previous book, *The Prostatitis Syndromes*, or my companion book to this one entitled, *Prostatitis and BPH*.

Prostate Biopsy

Often there is a knee-jerk reaction to biopsy the prostate if the PSA level is elevated or because a lump is felt on the prostate, but caution is warranted. Moe and Larry would do well to consider whether they would do anything different if their biopsies proved to be positive for prostate cancer. One viable option for prostate cancer is to undergo watchful waiting, either because the odds are that the tumor is small and slow growing, or because the treatments for prostate cancer are too drastic for men to consider.

Biopsies are done with transrectal ultrasound guidance. The ultrasound probe is placed in the rectum. A biopsy gun is threaded through the ultrasound probe. When the gun is fired a needle pokes through the wall of the rectum into the prostate. Using the ultrasound machine to guide the process, the doctor takes several samples from the prostate; the typical number of samples used to be six, but taking more is becoming common.

You might think that going through the rectum sounds dangerous. Indeed, in some areas of the world, the

---

[51] Murphy JJ: Letters and phone calls with the author. February 4, 2001. Reprinted with signed, written permission.

prostate is biopsied through the skin between the anus and testicles (the perineum). The perineal method avoids puncturing the rectum and should be less likely to cause infections.

Why do doctors in the United States go through the rectum? For the most part, because it's easier. I could not find any studies that adequately compared the two approaches of doing biopsies in terms of patient acceptance or side effects.

There is considerable expertise involved in doing biopsies. Some physicians are better than others are and it takes both skill and the right equipment to do prostate biopsies in the most successful manner possible.

What I Would Do

If it someday comes to a biopsy for myself, there are only about five physicians in the world that I would let do it. I would probably insist that at least 8 to 12 cores be taken not 6, I would insist on a second opinion, and I would insist on sedation for the procedure.

Today's biopsy techniques provide very thin 1 mm cores of tissue for the pathologist to examine. Many cases are difficult to call cancer and are called "atypia" or PIN (prostate intraepithelial neoplasm). Both conditions suggest a high risk for prostate cancer but are not definitive enough for therapy.

Dr. Jonathan Epstein, the senior prostate cancer pathologist at John's Hopkins Medical Institute, informed me that if he were diagnosed he would definitely get a second opinion on his slides. "Diagnosing prostate cancer is subjective," he told me, "1.5 percent of the time men are switched from cancer to having benign disease upon a second opinion."[52]

---

[52] Epstein J: Telephone interview with the author July 24, 2000.

Risks

Biopsies can be dangerous. I have known several men whose prostates swelled shut after their biopsy making them unable to urinate. One man has had constant rectal pain and itching since his biopsy. Some men come down with incurable prostatitis after a biopsy.

Is there a financial motive to doing biopsies? One man wrote me about how eager his urologist was to biopsy him. He took a cynical look at the situation. He found that in 1999 there were approximately 600,000 prostate biopsies in the United States. Only about one-third were positive for prostate cancer. He noted that at an average of $1,500 per biopsy, this inaccurate procedure generates 900 million dollars per year for the medical industry. Perhaps what made him most angry was the attitude he sensed. He felt urologists were doing biopsies, and when negative, were sending men home with a hearty "Isn't life grand, you don't have prostate cancer." In his opinion, they were neglecting to medically treat the prostatitis or BPH that must be causing the elevated PSA level. "It's enough to make the coldest of hearts cry," he wrote me.[53]

Biopsy Side Effects

The side effects of biopsy can be serious. About half of men will have blood in their semen for days to weeks after a biopsy, and 25 percent of men will have blood in their urine. Either situation can, in rare cases, become long lasting. A few men, around 1 to 2 percent, will experience rectal bleeding.[54]

All patients will experience what urologists euphemistically call "discomfort." It's what you would probably call pain. Most will be given antibiotics to prevent

---

[53] Name Withheld. Letter to the author. May 10, 2000.

[54] Rietbergen JBW, Kruger AEB, Kranse R, and Schröder FH: Complications of transrectal ultrasound-guided systematic sextant biopsies of the prostate: Evaluation of complication rates and risk factors within a population-based screening program. UROLOGY. 1997;49:875-880.

prostatitis, but this is not always successful. Because biopsies are typically done through the rectum, the prostate is exposed to rectal bacteria, and about 5 percent of men will develop fever or prostatitis, or will become sick with bacteria in their bloodstream. As noted, a few men (less than 1 percent) will be unable to urinate after a biopsy.

A patient who is without symptoms and perfectly healthy going into biopsy because of an elevated PSA may end up with serious temporary or permanent complications. While writing this book, I learned of an 80-year-old man who was biopsied for cancer and remains permanently catheterized as a side effect. He did not have cancer, and even if he had, it's unlikely that he would have undergone treatment at his age. He should not have been biopsied in the first place, in my opinion.

Another man complained bitterly to me about the pain of his biopsy and wondered what the "wisdom" was on anesthesia for biopsies.

The Real Risks from Prostatic Biopsies

I am generally amazed at how under-reported the side effects of surgical procedures can be. I did find one prospective study that tried to evaluate the true incidence of side effects after TRUS biopsy.[55] In 128 men, anything that required hospitalization was considered a major complication, and there was only one: a man who fainted and had seizures during his biopsy. All 128 men experienced "discomfort" with 25.4 percent of them experiencing moderate or severe "discomfort." I have noticed how studiously the word "pain" is avoided in some biopsy studies, which might lead you to ask your doctor how moderate or severe discomfort can occur without pain.

---

[55] Rodríguez LV and Terris MK: Risks and Complications of Transrectal Ultrasound Guided Prostate Needle Biopsy: A Prospective Study and Review of the Literature. *Journal of Urology.* 1998;160:2115-2120.

Slightly over five percent of the patients had fainting spells so significant that they dropped their systolic blood pressure below 90 (normal is 120). Just over eight percent of the patients had moderate or severe rectal bleeding, and seventy-one percent of the patients had moderate to severe bloody urine.

Delayed complications were defined as those lasting for three to seven days or more. Forty-seven percent of the men continued to have bloody urine, thirteen percent of men continued to have unspecified pain, 11.6 percent had trouble urinating, 9.9 percent had bloody stools, 9.1 percent had bloody semen, 9.1 percent had pain with urination, 3.3 percent had pain with bowel movements, and 2.5 percent had chills while 1.7 percent had fever despite the use of antibiotics for the procedure.

Interestingly, 19 percent of these 129 men (15%) said they wouldn't undergo a biopsy again without anesthesia. Your urologist may say that you will only feel a little pinch, but before the procedure is over you may wonder how a urologist's concept of a "little pinch" could be so different from your own. One man wrote me his biopsy was painful and that he "hurt like everything" all the way home. If he ever had a biopsy again, he said, it would be under sedation or anesthesia.

The Biopsy May Miss

Moe and Larry are surprised to find out that it's very easy for the biopsy needle to miss prostate cancer. Even if a doctor goes in multiple times with the needle to obtain cores, depending on the size of the prostate and the size of the cores, the amount sampled usually represents less than 1 percent of the prostate's tissue. Disease, including cancer, can easily be present in the 99 percent of the prostate that is not being sampled.

Urologists often do a "sextant" biopsy, sampling the prostate with six different needle sticks. One study that looked at men with PSA levels over 4 showed that prostatic biopsies found only 79 percent of the cancers on the first pass. The other 21 percent of the cancers were found only after the second, third, fourth, or even fifth biopsy was done.[56] All told, even with two separate "sextant" biopsy procedures the chance of identifying prostate cancer when it is present is only around 95 percent.

Pathologists

Moe and Larry need to consider who their pathologist will be. Most men don't even think to question who their pathologist is and they assume their pathology report is 100 percent accurate. You should always have your biopsy slide reviewed by an expert in prostate cancer pathology. These super-specialists are the "final word" on what grade your cancer is, or whether you really have cancer at all.

Special attention should be paid to the subspecialty of the pathologist. Are his or her special interests breast cancer or lung cancer, but not prostate cancer? Remember that your urologist or hospital may have contracted out the pathology work. They may have done so to the cheapest or most convenient, not the best. Even your urologist may not have any input into who reads the prostate biopsy slides. And your urologist may not know any more about the situation than you do.

The thin-needle-core biopsy is a recent innovation in prostate cancer biopsies. Most pathologists were trained before this technique was invented. For this reason, and for many other reasons, the presence of cancer and its Gleason grade and score may vary significantly between two pathologists reading the same slides. Rarely, when prostate cancer is diagnosed, surgery is done, and the final pathology will reveal that no prostate cancer was ever present. This is a disaster for each poor man that it

---

[56] Keetch, David W, Catalona William J, and Deborah S. Smith: Serial Prostatic Biopsies in Men with Persistently Elevated Serum Prostate Specific Antigen Values. *Journal of Urology.* June 1994: Vol. 151, 1571-1574.

happens to. The opposite can also occur. One hospital admitted in April 1999 that they missed misdiagnosed 19 men in the mid 1990s, telling them that they did not have prostate cancer, when in fact their biopsy slides should have been read positive for cancer. Men should consider having their prostate slides sent out for a second opinion to a recognized prostate cancer specialist. Reading biopsy slides is a complex and difficult process in which no one pathologist can be 100 percent accurate.

Moe and Larry's Biopsies

Moe and Larry decide to undergo biopsies. But first they make sure that their slides will be read at their local hospital and then also sent to a prostate cancer super-specialist for a second reading. They also make sure that DNA ploidy analysis (another important test) will be done. They also make sure that some tissue is banked in case they need a prostate cancer vaccine someday.

Moe underwent a biopsy and his prostate cancer was found to contain mostly Gleason grade 3, while Gleason grade 2 was less commonly present. He was assigned a Gleason score of 5 and was told to report his score to others as the equation "3 + 2 = 5" because it reveals all this information. Larry also underwent a biopsy. His results were 3 + 4 = 7.

An important issue for the man just diagnosed with prostate cancer is distinguishing the common slow-growing kind of prostate cancer from the more rare fast-growing type. Until a way to make this distinction definitively is discovered, the PSA test, Gleason score, and DNA ploidy status can help. Keep your eyes open for the latest and greatest tests that might distinguish fast-growing cancer from slow-growing cancer.

Look for Prostatitis in Your Biopsy

It's amazing how frequently prostatitis is seen in prostate cancer biopsies, but not reported to men. Many doctors apparently think it's not important for men to know about it. Prostatitis in biopsies is so common that many pathologists routinely don't even mention the finding in their report. This is inappropriate. There is prostatitis in one-half or more of men who are biopsied for prostate cancer, depending on how carefully it is looked for. You should be told! The pathologist doesn't report prostatitis in Moe and Larry's biopsies, and like most men, they never inquire about it, or ask if it was looked for.

A Better Way Than a Biopsy

One might think that a better way to screen for prostate cancer than undergoing an invasive biopsy would be to undergo prostatic massage, and have the prostatic fluid examined for the presence of prostate cancer cells. Spanish researchers have done exactly that; they found that looking for prostate cancer cells and other cytology had a predictive value for prostate cancer of 100%.[57]

Ask yourself if urologists are jumping on this new method of detecting prostate cancer as fast as they can. As a check for cancer, I'd rather undergo a prostatic massage than have needle stuck, multiple times, through my rectum and into my prostate to obtain a biopsy.

Biopsy to Treatment

Moe and Larry join as many support groups as they can. They join Us TOO International, Patient Advocates for Advanced Cancer Treatments (PAACT), The Education Center for Prostate Cancer Patients (ECPCP), The American

---

[57] Varo Solis C, Hens Perez A, Bachiller Burgos J, Figueroa Murillo E: [Prostatic exfoliative cytology obtained from urine samples after massage. Initial results]. *Actas Urol Esp.* 2002 Jun;26(6):398-406.

Prostate Society, and Man to Man. Armed with their PSA levels, Gleason scores, DRE results, and other test results, they go to as many meetings as they can. They also join the Internet *Prostate Problems Mailing List* (PPML), the *Patient to Physician Mailing List* (P2P), and are lucky enough to be invited onto the members only *Skunkworks Prostate Cancer Mailing List*. They also post to the Internet newsgroup sci.med.prostate.cancer. They read all the books they can about prostate cancer. Moe and Larry also get opinions from several different urologists, radiation oncologists, oncologists, cryosurgeons, and other patients.

Predictive Tables

It's time for Moe and Larry to try to predict how serious their prostate cancer might be. In fact, an important new tool in prostate cancer is the development of predictive tables that help men grasp the odds on the extent of prostate cancer. Dr. Alan Partin, at Johns Hopkins (a medical center in Baltimore, Maryland), created the first predictive tables. The predictive tables have become so important that, in my view, it is malpractice not to utilize them prior to treatment. Moe goes to the Partin Tables and plugs in his PSA of 8.0, his clinical stage of T1(c), and his Gleason score of 5.

The Partin tables tell Moe that his prostate cancer has a 75 percent change of being confined to his prostate, the probability of seminal vesicle extension is only 23 percent, and the probability of lymph node invasion is 0 percent.

Larry plugs in his information of a PSA of 16, clinical stage T2(a), and a Gleason score of 7. He is given only a 20 percent chance that his cancer is confined to his prostate, risk of extra-prostatic extension is 49 percent, seminal vesicle invasion 16 percent, and lymph node invasion 14 percent.

Larry breathes in sharply in disbelief. He was hoping the odds would be more in his favor. "I'm going to have to treat my cancer more aggressively than you treat yours," he tells Moe.

Doctors created the Partin tables by collecting PSA levels, clinical stages, and Gleason scores of over 4,000 men from three major medical centers. This information was then compared to the surgical pathology results after radical prostatectomy. One caveat is that there were not enough African-American men in the study, thus to use the tables for such men, and other ethnic groups, is questionable.

Moe and Larry, with their doctor's help, use other predictive tables besides the Partin Tables. They also use the Narayan Tables and the Bluestein Tables. All these predictive tables help them to realize what the extent of their prostate cancer might be.

The ProstaScint Scan

ProstaScint is the trade name for a scanning technique for prostate cancer that may help to tell whether prostate cancer has spread to the lymph nodes. It can be used prior to definitive treatment to decide if cancer is localized to the prostate. Men are scanned after receiving an injection of radioactive labeled antibody, and also scanned a second time between four and seven days later. The worst part of the test for many men is the bowel prep that they must take to clear out their intestines before being scanned. I found the most current list of places that perform the ProstaScint scan to be on the Internet at www.prostascint.com.

Diagnostic Laparotomy and Lymph Node Biopsy

Another tool for staging prostate cancer is the diagnostic laparotomy. The laparoscope is like a long, thin telescope. By poking a hole in the abdomen, the doctor can thread the laparoscope inside and see the pelvic lymph nodes. The nodes can be biopsied. If they are positive, the cancer has already spread outside the prostate. Conventional wisdom eliminates the radical prostatectomy as an option if this is the case.

Bone Scan

The bone scan is currently the most sensitive test for detecting if prostate cancer has spread to the bones. Unfortunately, it's not sensitive enough. The cancer in the bones has to become large enough for the bone scan to pick it up. A negative bone scan suggests that the cancer has not spread to the bones but does not rule it out completely, because many metastases are too small to be seen with a bone scan, resulting in a false negative scan. Bone scans only pick up large-enough-to-detect disease.

MRI with Endorectal Coil

Magnetic resonance imaging (MRI) is a way to take very good pictures of the inside of the human body using magnetic fields. Moe and Larry will be placed inside big magnet to have their MRIs done. Better pictures of the prostate can be obtained by placing a probe (endorectal coil) in the rectum.

Moe and Larry undergo MRI with endorectal coil. The skill in using the endorectal coil device, and in reading the results of the pictures; however, varies with the experience of the examiner and the institution. Moe and Larry both go to an institution where the procedure is done often, and where the radiologists are highly skilled at reading the results.

There is a growing body of evidence that MRI with endorectal coil gives superior images of the prostate and seminal vesicles, and you should probably prefer one to a regular MRI. Certainly, when I look at the images personally, I see clearer, sharper and more detailed images with MRI with endorectal coil.

MRI with endorectal coil can be difficult to get. As I write this, according to General Electric who makes the machines, there is not a machine with an endorectal coil in Chicago. The University of California at San Francisco, and Sloan-Kettering in New York both do MRI with endorectal coil. In fact, those places and others are cooperating on a study of endorectal coil and spectroscopy together for prostate cancer patients. Watch for the results of that study.

Bad Prognostic Signs

Cancer that has spread outside of the prostate is bad news. "Margin positive disease" means that when the prostate and surrounding tissue from surgery are examined cancer is found in the margins. Therefore, cancer was left behind.

Patients with margin positive disease, or positive lymph nodes, or invasion of cancer into the seminal vesicles do poorly; the survival curves for margin-positive disease and lymph node-positive disease are poor compared to those of men with organ-confined disease.[58] This discouraging prognosis is the reason so much effort is invested prior to making treatment decisions to find out whether prostate cancer is completely contained within the prostate.

One study found that odds of ten-year survival were 75 percent when prostate cancer is confined to the prostate, 55 percent when there is local spread outside the prostate, and only 15 percent when there are distant metastases.[59]

Find out about your pathology report after your radical prostatectomy. Look for these technical terms: focal extra-capsular extension, established extra-capsular

---

[58] Paulson DF: Impact of radical prostatectomy in the management of clinically localized disease. *Journal of Urology.* 1994;152:1826-1830.

[59] Woolf, Steven H, MD, MPH: Screening for Prostate Cancer with Prostate-Specific Antigen. *New England Journal of Medicine.* 1995;333(21):1401-1405.

extension, seminal vesicle invasion, or positive pelvic lymph nodes.

Localized Prostate Cancer

Most or all of the tests above are done, and it appears that Moe and Larry have localized prostate cancer. This book concentrates on treating clinically localized prostate cancer, because that is the most commonly diagnosed type today.

Watchful Waiting for Localized Prostate Cancer

The first thing I would do if I were diagnosed with prostate cancer would be to begin watchful waiting for a period of weeks, months, or even years. The second thing I would do is start active non-invasive therapy (ANIT), which I will explain in the next chapter.

WATCHFUL WAITING DOES NOT MEAN DOING NOTHING! Please scream this in the ear of every man you meet at prostate cancer support groups. I have seen men fail to understand this concept hundreds of times. *Watchful waiting is a form of treatment* and in fact, it may be the best treatment for many, even most men, with localized prostate cancer.

Classically, watchful waiting means watching your prostate cancer until it causes symptoms—if it ever does—and then treating the symptoms.

In older days, if bone pain occurred from metastatic cancer, men would be treated with castration or estrogen. Blocking male hormones by these methods usually helped to slow down or stop prostate cancer. If urinary blockage occurred despite castration or estrogen, it was treated with transurethral resection of the prostate (TURP).

More recently, treating with medications that block the male hormones (medical hormone blockade) instead of castration has come into being. Watchful waiting has evolved and improved like every other form of prostate cancer therapy.

You will not be alone if you chose watchful waiting. Not long ago, it was estimated that about one-third of all men with prostate cancer chose watchful waiting, about one-third chose surgery, and about one-third chose radiation therapy in some form.

Always remember that the least harmful treatment for prostate cancer, the one that interrupts your life the least, and is appropriate if your cancer is small and slow-growing (which we never know with 100 percent certainty), is watchful waiting. Watchful waiting preserves your sexuality and urinary continence; the treatment itself does not harm you, unless your cancer becomes symptomatic and you must start hormone blockade or have a TURP.

Men who chose watchful waiting do so because the odds are often high that they have slow-growing prostate cancer that will never affect them. They expect, and hope, to live their lives and eventually die from some other problem—not prostate cancer.

Question Your Doctor

One of the most serious complaints that men have against urologists is that they only tell men about radical surgery, as if it were the only option. Question whatever your doctor tells you. Many men have never, in all their lives, questioned a doctor, but with prostate cancer everything is debatable and the data is often lacking, woefully deficient, or biased. Get a second, third, fourth, and even fifth opinion. You must decide for yourself what is right for you. Radical surgery is not the only option, in fact, based on controlled scientific studies, and independent studies of side effects, the radical prostatectomy is never an option for the man who wants to extend his life and maintain quality of life.

Watchful Waiting

In reality, it can be argued that the vast majority of all men with prostate cancer "choose" watchful waiting because so many men who have prostate cancer never know they have it. Most men around the world never undergo a rectal exam or receive a PSA test, so they never know they have prostate cancer. In addition, many men who do get tested have prostate cancer too small for tests to detect.

Watchful waiting is an option because most prostate cancer is small and slow-growing, and because many men are older when they are diagnosed with prostate cancer. For example, one review paper found that the average age of diagnosis of prostate cancer was 72 years of age, that the average life expectancy for men was 74.2 years, and that the average age of death from prostate cancer was 77 years. These numbers mean that most men die of other causes before their prostate cancer has a chance to kill them.[60]

The majority of men with prostate cancer today feel fine by conventional medical standards and will go on to live their lives without ever dying from prostate cancer. They will die *with* prostate cancer inside them, but not *from* it. They will die from heart attacks, strokes, lung disease, and many other problems instead of their prostate cancer.

No randomized controlled study acceptable to me has ever shown that any prostate cancer treatment works better than watchful waiting. Yet, the prostate cancer world is replete with doctors and patients who advocate treatments that immediately decrease the quality of a man's life. In short, the treatment for prostate cancer is often worse than the disease. If you can get away without damaging treatment you come out ahead.

In one study from JAMA, the authors observe:

> "Once prostate cancer is diagnosed and treated, the patient's life is necessarily and permanently altered. Even if he is thought to be cured, his level of functioning may be diminished, and he may sustain specific complications of treatment, such as impotence, urinary incontinence, or bowel dysfunction. He

---

[60] Sandhu SS and Kaisary AV: Localized carcinoma of the prostate: a paradigm of uncertainty. *Postgraduate Medical Journal.* 1997;73:691-696.

is also likely to suffer negative psychosocial and economic consequences from having cancer."[61]

Watchful waiting is a difficult choice for many men. The natural response to cancer is "Oh my God, I must do something immediately." But prostate cancer is not a "conventional" cancer. Only a small proportion of all men with prostate cancer die from it.

As a society we have a knee-jerk, primitive, and wrong-headed belief that all prostate cancer must be cut out, irradiated or poisoned. Support groups all across the nation are full of men who made hasty, aggressive, treatment decisions and will be suffering the consequences for the rest of their lives. Men who have suffered treatment disasters often encourage those newly diagnosed to be better informed than they themselves were before making a treatment decision.

Studies of Watchful Waiting

What happens to men who undergo watchful waiting, men who wait until symptoms appear and then undergo treatment—hormone blockade or TURP—as necessary? To find out, I researched the medical literature for important studies addressing this question. I begin the summary of each study with the year in which it was published.

1988: In Edinburgh, Scotland between 1977 and 1987, 69 men, average age 74, were diagnosed with prostate cancer based on seeing it in prostate chips removed during transurethral resection of the prostate (TURP) for benign prostatic hyperplasia (BPH). The probability of being alive

---

[61] Litwin, Mark, MD, MPH; Ron D. Hays, PhD; Arlene Fink, PhD; Patricia A. Ganz, MD; Barbara Leake, PhD; Gary E. Leach, MD; and Robert H. Brook, MD, ScD: Quality-of-Life Outcomes in Men Treated for Localized Prostate Cancer. JAMA. January 11, 1995: Vol 273 (No. 2) p. 129. Copyright 1995 by the American Medical Association. Quoted with signed, written permission.

after 5 years was only 50 percent in this group of 69 men, but only six men (8.6 percent) died of prostate cancer during the study; most men died of something else.[62]

1988: In Manchester, England 120 men, average age 74.8, diagnosed with prostate cancer between 1980 and 1986 were studied for 7 years.[63] All the men had negative bone scans, so their prostate cancer was confined to the prostate according to tests available at the time. Ninety percent of the men in the study had symptoms such as urinary trouble (today most men diagnosed with prostate cancer don't have any symptoms). Only five of the 120 men (4 percent) died of prostate cancer during the 7-year study period. Forty-eight other men (40 percent) died during the 7-year period from diseases unrelated to prostate cancer, which means that the men were 10 times as like to die of something else than their prostate cancer.

1992: Of 122 men in Sweden, average age 68, with low or medium-grade localized prostate cancer followed for an average of 7.6 years with watchful waiting, only 9 men (7 percent) died of prostate cancer while 38 men (31 percent) died of other causes.[64]

1994: In Sweden, from March 1977 to February 1984, 117 men with localized prostate cancer (stages T1-T2), were placed on watchful waiting. Over the next 12.5 years, only 11 (9 percent) of them died of prostate cancer while 74 (63 percent) died of something else.[65] The critique

---

[62] Goodman CM, Busuttil A, and Chisholm GD: Age, and Size and Grade of Tumour Predict Prognosis in Incidentally Diagnosed Carcinoma of the Prostate. *British Journal of Urology.* 1988;62:576-580.

[63] George NJR: Natural History of Localized Prostate Cancer Managed by Conservative Therapy Alone. *The Lancet.* 1988:494-497.

[64] Adolfsson J, Carstensen J, Lowhagen T: Deferred treatment in clinically localised prostatic carcinoma. *British Journal of Urology.* 1992 Feb;69(2):183-7.

[65] Johansson JE: Watchful Waiting for Early Stage Prostate Cancer. UROLOGY. 1994;43(2):138-142.

of this study is that many of the men in the study were around 75 years of age, while younger men are being diagnosed with prostate cancer today.

1994: In a pooled analysis of 828 men from previous watchful waiting studies with an average age of 69,[66] some very interesting results were obtained. The 10-year prostate cancer-specific survival for men with low-grade prostate cancer was 87 percent. The 10-year survival for men with medium-grade prostate cancer was also 87 percent. The 10-year survival for men with high-grade prostate cancer was only 34 percent. So you can see that over 10 years, watchful waiting has a very good outcome in terms of survival for most men, as most men have low and medium-grade prostate cancer.

In this study, younger men did better than older men. This is important because there may be an erroneous assumption floating around in the prostate cancer world that younger men always have more aggressive prostate cancers. Of all the men with low and medium-grade prostate cancer that were *under age 61*, their 10-year prostate cancer-specific survival was 97 percent. Of the men with low and medium-grade cancer *over age 61*, their 10-year prostate cancer-specific survival dipped to 84 percent.

One explanation for this is that prostate cancer is simply being discovered earlier in its course than it used to be, but the nature of low and medium grade prostate cancer remains the same; it usually grows slowly as men age.

1997: One of the best studies ever done on watchful waiting came out of Sweden and was published in the

---

[66] Chodak GW, Thisted RA, Gerber GS, Johansson JE, Adolfsson J, Jones GW, Chisholm GD, Moskovitz B, Livne PM, and Warner J: Results of conservative management of clinically localized prostate cancer. *New England Journal of Medicine.* 1994;330:242-248.

Journal of the American Medical Association.[67] Two-hundred and twenty-three men underwent watchful waiting. The average age of the men in the study was 72. The first thing to note was that only 5.9 percent of the men lived for 15 years. The second thing is that only 11 percent of the men died from prostate cancer. This study certainly points out the favorable odds for watchful waiting in the older population—virtually 90 percent of the deaths that occurred were believed to be from causes other than prostate cancer.

2000: A Florida study looked at 54 men, average age 76, with clinically localized diagnosed prostate cancer between 1991 and 1998, who elected to undergo watchful waiting. The average follow-up time was four years. In that time only 3 of the 76 men developed metastases and presumably only those three men are at risk of dying from their prostate cancer in the near future.[68]

When Prostate Cancer Kills

The previous studies show that watchful waiting does well for two reasons: 1) most prostate cancer is slow-growing and, 2) most men die of something else before prostate cancer kills them.

These facts are not comforting to the men who actually die from prostate cancer. The conventional advice given by urologists today is that if you have more than a 10-year lifespan, you need to be treated for prostate cancer. Is that advice correct?

If you look at only men who live 10 years or longer after the diagnosis of prostate cancer, the disease appears

---

[67] Jan-Erik Johansson, Lars Holmberg, Sara Johannson, Reinhold Bergström, and Hans-Olov Adami: Fifteen Year Survival in Prostate Cancer: A Prospective, Population-Based Study in Sweden. JAMA. 1997;277(6):467-471.

[68] Neulander EZ, Duncan RC, Tiguert R, Posey JT, and Soloway MS: Deferred treatment of localized prostate cancer in the elderly: the impact of the age and stage at the time of diagnosis on the treatment decision. *BJU International.* 2000;85:699-704.

more lethal. In one study of 65 men who lived for at least 10 years after their diagnosis of prostate cancer, more than half—63 percent—died from prostate cancer.[69]

But the nature of prostate cancer is very important. Just because men are diagnosed at a younger age today with the PSA test does not necessarily mean that they have more aggressive prostate cancer. In fact in the pooled analysis of 828 watchful waiting patients, those men under age 61 with stage T1 or T2 prostate cancer had the highest metastasis-free survival following watchful waiting. Men under age 61 had 97 percent metastasis free survival at 10 years, which was the best survival of any subgroup.[70]

On the other hand the very fact that prostate cancer can be picked up in younger men at all may mean that they have a more aggressive form of prostate cancer—some studies, and urologists, have suggested this.

I am suspicious of this self-serving conclusion! Urologists who are publishing these studies say that younger men with prostate cancer, prime surgical candidates because they are essentially healthy, are the ones who benefit from radical surgery. If all the studies showed that, I might believe them, but they don't. Since the quality of the studies are poor, and the nature of such studies are so pro-surgery, I remain skeptical, and you should too.

The bottom line is that many men who chose watchful waiting will never have significant symptoms from their prostate cancer and will never suffer side effects from treating their prostate cancer in a harmful manner. The same man for whom watchful waiting is great for at age 75, might have his prostate cancer picked up at 55 today, and might undergo the side effects of unnecessary treatment for 20 years for nothing!

---

[69] Aus G, Hugosson J, Norlen L: Long-term survival and mortality in prostate cancer treated with noncurative intent. *Journal of Urology.* 1995;154(2 Pt. 1):460-465.
[70] Chodak GW: The Role of Watchful Waiting in the Management of Localized Prostate Cancer. *Journal of Urology.* 1994;152:1766-1768.

Young Men and Watchful Waiting

I must talk more about the young man conundrum, because I am so concerned about it.

One school of conventional wisdom is that watchful waiting is a good choice for older men with low-grade prostate cancer (Gleason scores 2, 3, 4). Statistically, such men—especially if older in age—are likely to die of some other cause before their cancer becomes aggressive enough to kill them. The average age at which prostate cancer is diagnosed is 72, and only 47 percent of 72-year-old men live 10 more years. Thus the view that watchful waiting is best way to preserve the quality of life in such men, rather than to intervene with harmful therapy.

But don't swallow the "Watchful waiting is for old men only" theory whole. Watchful waiting could be best for younger men, and other less harmful therapies than radical surgery could be even better.

If 50-year-old men have small cancers or incidental cancers discovered by the PSA test, it's quite possible that the best thing to do for their quality of life is to watch the cancer until their PSA rises to a certain level, or until their cancer progresses locally, and then to put them on hormone blockade. It's quite possible that young men treated this way would have the greatest quality of life and life expectancy—the best outcome—of any prostate cancer treatment. Or perhaps hormone blockade followed by Proscar maintenance would be the best treatment, or cryotherapy, or radiation seed implants. There are many options. It's also possible that a true cure will be found within 10 years.

Young men who undergo surgery are being asked to endure the side effects of treatment for 10 years or longer, before any survival benefit kicks in, if it ever does. They might have to wait 15 or 20 years for a survival benefit of 1 year to kick in! These scenarios are not appealing to me.

We need quality studies to know the best treatment for sure. There is a lot of soul searching to do. A 1993 analysis found no benefit for the radical prostatectomy or radiation therapy versus watchful waiting for patients with clinically localized prostate cancer.[71]

Many studies focus on death (mortality) and completely ignore quality of life issues. One study measured the quality of life in prostate cancer patients and found that, overall; men without treatment had a better quality of life than those who underwent aggressive treatment:

> "Even after controlling for the sexual and urinary dysfunction experienced by older men without cancer, those receiving therapeutic interventions [like surgery or radiation] for their prostate cancer were found to have poorer disease-targeted HRQOL [Health-related Quality of Life]."[72]

The Watchful Waiting Game

It's very hard to explain the lies, damn lies, and statistics to men when it comes to prostate cancer. But there is definitely a "game" being played when it comes to surgery versus watchful waiting. For a moment let's only think about 100 men who all have lethal prostate cancer. Lethal prostate cancer is a minority of all prostate cancer, but we can't get around the fact that 7.5 percent of men with prostate cancer are going to die from it. I want to give you a likely timeline for men with deadly prostate cancer.

---

[71] Fleming, C, Wasson JH, Albertson PC: A Decision Analysis of Alternative Treatment Strategies for Clinically Localized Prostate Cancer. JAMA. 1993;269;2650-2658.

[72] Litwin, Mark, MD, MPH; Ron D. Hays, PhD; Arlene Fink, PhD; Patricia A. Ganz, MD; Barbara Leake, PhD; Gary E. Leach, MD; and Robert H. Brook, MD, ScD: Quality-of-Life Outcomes in Men Treated for Localized Prostate Cancer. JAMA. January 11, 1995:273(2);129. Copyright 1995 by the American Medical Association. Quoted with signed, written permission.

Birth----→Death from prostate cancer.

Now, I am going to add a few more details to the timeline from birth to death from prostate cancer:

Birth → prostate cancer starts → prostate cancer spreads on microscopic level → PSA test is positive → DRE examination → Death from prostate cancer.

What I want you to understand is that the PSA test may be too late. It may be picking up prostate cancer after metastases start for many, most, or even all men. We don't know for sure. Therefore, if this scenario is true, picking up deadly prostate cancer by the digital rectal exam is too late, and picking up deadly cancer by the PSA is too late; it's already out of the prostate.

Where has PSA testing moved us? Earlier in the time line no doubt, but if the prostate cancer is the aggressive type, has prostate cancer already escaped the prostate? If so, PSA testing really makes no difference, but; AND THIS IS THE IMPORTANT POINT, studies can be made to look as if it does.

We don't know where PSA testing has moved us on the time line in regards to metastatic disease. Urologists have the most self-interest to believe PSA testing has moved us to a beneficial point on the timeline, but unfortunately, controlled studies have not proved that it has done so, at least not in a way that increases survival. This is the dilemma—the uncertainty—facing all us men.

Watchful waiting is a reasonable starting point for all men with small, low-grade prostate cancers until a controlled study proves otherwise. In fact, there are those that believe it is the best option for such men.

Pluses

The pluses for watchful waiting are numerous. If you chose watchful waiting and your cancer never ends up bothering you, then you also never get harmed by aggressive prostate cancer treatments. You get to enjoy life with intact sexuality, urinary continence, and without bowel problems—just to name a few possible side effects with other treatments. It may also be possible that the "wonder cure" will be found during your period of watchful waiting. Watchful waiting gives you time to learn about prostate cancer—and you need it—because it's a complicated and controversial disease.

What I Think

I am not one of those people who think that nothing should be done for prostate cancer. I am a proponent of early diagnosis of prostate cancer and extensive prostate cancer education. I am in favor of mobilizing research and finding out how to cure and prevent prostate cancer. I am in favor of making the best possible decision. What I am against is doing something harmful and ineffective, just to be doing something, but more on that in the upcoming chapters.

Guilt Factor

Watchful waiting involves a high guilt factor. If men go on watchful waiting and it fails for them, then they and their doctor feel a great deal of guilt and often wish they had chosen a more radical treatment. Those who continue to read this book should feel less guilty about watchful waiting—and start to see it as sometimes being very rational.

I met a man who was probably a perfect candidate for watchful waiting. He insisted upon getting a radical prostatectomy even against his urologist's advice. He was nearly 80 years old and had no symptoms from his prostate cancer. He doctor-shopped until he found a urologist who would take out his prostate. Now he has serious side effects from his surgery. This man preaches to other men about the benefits of surgery, yet it is uncertain that he received any benefit from surgery, and clearly he was hurt by it.

Why don't more men chose watchful waiting—especially older men with low-grade cancers? I think many men don't understand that the statistics are generally favorable for watchful waiting. It seems to be difficult for many men to "wait" when they have cancer, which is partly due to a lack of understanding about the disease and its treatments. It's also part of the American way to be aggressive in treating cancer, despite the evidence that we are often too aggressive with prostate cancer. It's also hard for doctors to encourage watchful waiting for fear the cancer will spread and they will be sued.

Urologist Thomas Stamey says:

> "I believe that when the final chapter of this disease is written, which is unlikely to be in my lifetime, never in the history of oncology will so many men have been so overtreated for one disease."[73]

---

[73] Stamey, Thomas. Perspectives on Prostate Cancer Diagnosis and Treatment: A Roundtable. UROLOGY. 2001:58;135-141. Quoted with permission.

Active Non-Invasive Therapy (ANIT)

If I had prostate cancer, I would begin watchful waiting, but the second thing I would do, would be to begin active non-invasive therapy (ANIT).

The term "active non-invasive therapy" was coined by prostate cancer survivor Sandy Goldman. It means doing everything healthy, and avoiding drastic and harmful measures, while still treating your prostate cancer.

I read about Sandy on the internet when he said, "To all those who gave me . . . the fortitude to say 'no' to urologists who wanted to cut, cut, cut, I say 'thank you'. . . . Watchful Waiting? Phooey. I'm not 'waiting' for anything except for the sun to rise tomorrow and to see it happen! I now call it [the pro-active regimen] Active Non-Invasive Therapy (ANIT)."

Sandy Goldman provided a better term for the next step beyond watchful waiting by coining the phrase "active non-invasive therapy."

ANIT Means

Active non-invasive therapy means following your prostate cancer with prostate specific antigen (PSA) tests and digital rectal exams (DREs). It means taking up the study of prostate cancer by reading books, searching the Internet, and joining groups such as Us TOO International, Patient Advocates for Advanced Cancer Treatments, and the Education Center for Prostate Cancer Patients. It means trying to decide how to use the latest advances in predicting the course of prostate cancer. It means becoming politically active in support of prostate cancer research. And it means reducing stress and living a healthier lifestyle.

Pat Flynn Story

The first time it was checked, Fifty-seven year old Pat Flynn's PSA was 2.9. The following year it rose to 4.1. His urologist suggested a biopsy, which hurt, but there was no cancer.

The following year Pat's PSA jumped to 7.5. He was prescribed the antibiotic ciprofloxacin to treat prostatitis, which may have been caused by his biopsy the year before. The PSA went down to 5.7, which was not judged to be enough of a decline.

Pat underwent a second biopsy, "They really hurt me," he lamented. The second biopsy was positive for prostate cancer in ten percent of one of six samples that were taken. His Gleason score was 3 + 3 = 6.

"My urologist recommended that I have a radical prostatectomy in the near future, but I should investigate all the options," Pat said.

Pat discovered a lot by researching on his own. "I got very active in checking into prostate cancer and talked to a lot of men who were dealing with my dilemma and I decided to change my lifestyle and monitor my PSA every four months. I've come to believe that the number of men in their 50's and 60's that have prostate cancer cells in their prostate is in the millions, yet only 30,000 actually die from the cancer. Most die from something else like heart disease while having the cancer cells in them."

Pat mentioned that he has a libido that he cares about, and that he went to prostate cancer support groups where he discovered unfortunate men who suffered disturbing adverse side effects from their prostate cancer treatments.

"Men who have the radical prostatectomy are very defensive about what they did being the right thing. They don't want to admit that they may have made a mistake.

They think the operation saved their lives. The same with cryosurgery and radiation," Pat said.

"I really feel for those men. Had I not checked things out, I might have suffered their fate. I might even be doing the wrong action here, but I believe in what I'm doing," Pat said with great passion.

Pat changed his lifestyle. He started exercising, he reduced his stress and started meditating, he changed his diet including avoiding red meat, and he started taking vitamins and supplements. He also began checking his PSA every four months and it has gone steadily down, from 5.7 to 4.5, 3.5, 3.6, 2.6, and finally to 2.3, his latest result.

Pat is an example of a man doing ANIT. He changed his lifestyle, he eliminated stress, and his PSA has been going down.

The Rabon Ring and ANIT

There is a lot you can do to lower your PSA, and in doing so, probably lower your risk of prostate cancer. You need to change your lifestyle. One of your goals is to lower your PSA and stop the "leaky prostate" syndrome.

One of the worst things that men do is sit down, smashing their prostates on the chairs underneath them. Men, some would say, were meant to be hunters and warriors, not sedentary chair-jockeys. Sitting on our prostates all day, day after day, is not good for us.

I met the distinguished urologist Larry D. Rabon, MD, at a National Institutes of Health meeting on prostatitis. He presented a report that sitting on a doughnut cushion could lower the PSA level in men. I was impressed by his sincerity and data. He recommended a larger study, which would have been easy to do, but his urological colleagues apparently had no interest in doing one.

The Rabon Ring, an inflatable doughnut, is available from:

Larry Rabon, MD

Urology
306 South McQueen St.
Florence, SC 29501
tel: (843)665-2200
fax: (843)665-1911

A Styrofoam ring prostate cushion, called the Thera-Seat, is available from the Prostatitis Foundation's web site at, www.Prostatitis.org.

It's also easy to go out and buy a padded toilet seat, detach the padded ring from the cover, and throw it on your chair, so that it takes the pressure of your prostate when you sit. You can place a cloth or cover over it for aesthetic reasons. Sit on the ring for few weeks, or months, and see if your PSA goes down.

If you experience any side effects from sitting on a cushion, such as back pain, hip pain or other problems, stop using the device.

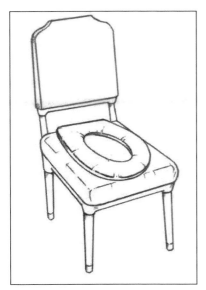

Figure 13. Sitting on doughnut cushion may lower your PSA. (Artist: Ramie Balbuena)

Diet and Exercise as Part of ANIT

In 2002, UCLA scientists took blood from 14 men who followed a low-fat diet and exercise program for 11 days. The scientists exposed prostate cancer cells to the men's blood. They found that prostate cancer cell growth was reduced by 30 percent after eleven days of diet and exercise.

The study suggests, what we probably know intuitively, that by being healthier you can enhance your body's ability to fight cancer. I could go on and on about diet and exercise, but I think those topics deserve their own book.

Viagra, Levitra, and Cialis as Part of ANIT

All men who can safely be put on Viagra, Levitra, or Cialis, and want to try one of these sex-enhancing drugs, should be started on one as part of active non-invasive therapy. These are sexual wonder drugs. By seeing how good your sex life can be, you will think more carefully before undergoing prostate cancer treatments that will destroy your sexual function, and you might make better choices.

Prostatitis and BPH

Prostatitis and BPH are the big imitators in prostate cancer, causing confusion. Independently of any cancer, prostatitis or BPH can raise the PSA. Unfortunately, the medical profession has neglected prostatitis, and even today, its cause and treatment often remain a mystery. As part of ANIT for your prostate cancer, I strongly suggest getting prostatitis and BPH diagnosed and treated in a non-surgical manner.

Summary of Several Things

As part of active non-invasive therapy, you should be kinder to your prostate and your body. You should stop crushing your prostate when you sit on it for hours and hours by using a ring cushion. You should start to diet and exercise to fight cancer. You should rid yourself of the stress in your life. You should get prostatitis and BPH diagnosed and treated, non-surgically. You should try out Viagra, Levitra, or Cialis to improve your sexual function. And, your prostate cancer should be followed with regular PSA tests and digital rectal exams. You should visit many doctors who are experts on prostate cancer treatments.

Charles Myers, MD

Snuffy Meyers, MD, a medical oncologist and prostate cancer survivor, has said:

> "In truth, if you have a Gleason 6 carcinoma or lower, and a PSA that's under 10, a very significant proportion of men in that group actually don't need to do anything other than diet and lifestyle."[74]

The Next Step

When should you jump from active non-invasive therapy to adding some other form of treatment? If I had a specific answer to that question for every man, I would deserve the Nobel Prize. The general answer is, though, if your PSA level is going up; more specifically, if it goes up three times in a row. Particularly if it goes up by more than 25 percent—which helps eliminate laboratory error. Also, be on guard, if you develop new symptoms, or if the digital rectal examination of your prostate changes for the worse.

---

[74] Meyers, Charles: A Presentation by Charles E. Myers Jr., MD, to the Kettering Medical Center Prostate Cancer Support Group on April 25, 2002. Available at: http://www.hormonerefractorypca.org/myers425.htm. Quoted with email permission from the author.

PC SPES

After watchful waiting and active non-invasive therapy, the next thing I would do if I had prostate cancer would be to start PC SPES. But will I be able to get it?

Mario Menelly, a manager at a utility company, had urinary trouble when he was 42 years old, but his physician denied him a PSA test. "Welcome to middle age, Mario," the physician said.

Mario endured another year with urinary symptoms. In September 1996, Mario went to the doctor again. His PSA was 100! He underwent a biopsy and all six biopsy samples showed evidence of cancer. His Gleason score was 9. There was evidence of perineural invasion, his cancer was aneuploid, tumors were present in his seminal vesicles on MRI, his ProstaScint scan was positive for abdominal lymph nodes. Mario had a death sentence. The only good news was that his bone scan was negative.

Mario went for five opinions and they were all highly pessimistic. He started on an organic diet and selenium. His PSA remained stable for 4 months, but by March 1997 it had risen to 122.0. Mario started taking a lot of vitamins and supplements. He had all his mercury amalgam fillings replaced. Then, he discovered PC SPES.

"The rest is history," Mario says. He started on nine capsules of PC SPES per day and in one month his PSA went from 122 to 11. He reduced his dosage to six capsules a day and his PSA continued to fall to 1. "My prostatic acid phosphatase (PAP) also declined, from 10 to 1, during this period," Mario told me.

Mario has found that his PSA will rise if he reduces his dosage of PC SPES too much. By 2000, Mario's PSA was 0.2 and he intended to maintain it at that level.

"All of my urinary symptoms are gone," Mario says, "And I no longer have any fatigue and I feel better than I have felt in years."

Side Effects

There are side effects from PC SPES. Mario Menelley suffered nipple tenderness for most of the first year on PC SPES and some breast enlargement. Because of the PC SPES he now has very little body hair on his legs, chest, and arms. His libido is way down, although he can still have intercourse and achieve orgasm. "Some men on PC SPES do reach the point of impotency," Mario warns.

Some men have reported blood clots when taking PC SPES. Taking aspirin may not prevent this serious side effect, as some men assume. Instead, another anticoagulant medication such as coumadin may be needed.

Paradoxically, a few men have had bleeding problems while on PC SPES. Side effects are why this product and other over-the-counter medications should be taken under the supervision of a knowledgeable physician.

Creation of PC SPES

PC SPES came about because a gynecologist was dying of metastatic prostate cancer. He had metastases to the lungs and pelvic area and had been given 6 months to live. He went to his sister-in-law, Dr. Sophie Chen, who had been doing laboratory research for five years on Chinese herbal preparations. She had previously worked for well-known drug companies such as Merck and Bayer. Dr. Chen and her brother-in-law had heard of Dr. Xuhui Wang in China, a medical doctor and ninth generation herbalist. They knew that he had an herbal preparation for prostate cancer.

Dr. Chen and her brother-in-law went to China to get the raw formula. Dr. Chen placed her brother-in-law's cancer cells in mice, where it grew. Using the mice as test subjects, Dr. Chen set up a series of experiments. She kept modifying the original formula to maximize prostate cancer death in the mice. She also tested her preparations against normal healthy human cells to makes sure it was not toxic. She remained skeptical because success in the laboratory does not always translate into success in people.

Finally, after about a year of work on the herbal combination, Dr. Chen's brother-in-law was allowed to take the preparation in 1992. After only 3 months his PSA went from 180 to less than 4, and over time it went even lower. After a year of being on PC SPES his bone scan started to clear up; the metastases were disappearing.

By 2000, still taking PC SPES, Dr. Chen's brother-in-law was alive and well without any signs of prostate cancer. Meanwhile, in 1996, a company called Botanic Lab, in Brea, California was set up to make PC SPES.

PC SPES is an over-the-counter combination of eight herbs—seven Chinese herbs along with the American herb saw palmetto. PC stands for prostate cancer and SPES is Latin for "hope." PC SPES means prostate cancer hope.

Action

PC SPES appears to have several mechanisms of action. Some studies show that it works like estrogen. The saw palmetto it contains probably blocks hormones at the level of the prostate. It is thought to have anti-oxidant and anti-inflammatory properties. Most importantly, PC SPES appears to have unique cancer killing properties, including a direct killing effect on prostate cancer.

Use Before Hormone Blockade?

PC SPES was on the way to being recommended as the first and best treatment for prostate cancer, before it fell from grace.

It should probably be used before double or triple hormone blockade, because it has fewer side effects than double or triple hormone blockade, and because once resistance to hormone blockade develops, PC SPES does not work as well, although it still works over half the time.

There are many, many success stories of men who chose to use PC SPES as their first therapy.

On the other hand, even if a man has been on hormone blockade and it fails, over half the time that man will still respond to PC SPES.

Side Effects

PC SPES can cause nipple tenderness, breast enlargement, nausea, diarrhea and a decrease in libido. It does not necessarily make you impotent—just decreases sexual desire. "The Plumbing can still be called on to perform if called to action," as one man describes it. Perhaps PC SPES's most serious side effect is that it sometimes causes blood clots. Men taking PC SPES may need to take blood thinners at the same time. For this reason, you should take PC SPES only under your doctor's supervision.

For the curious, the full list of ingredients of PC SPES includes *Scutellaria baicalensis, Glycyrrhiza glabra, Ganoderma lucidium, Isatis indigotica, Panax pseudo-ginseng, Serona repens* (saw palmetto), *Dendrantherma morifolium,* and *Rabdosia rubescens.*

The Fall of PC SPES

In 2002 the headlines screamed, "FDA Warning: Stop Taking PC SPES Immediately!"

The California Department of Health had tested PC SPES and found it to contain sodium warfarin (Coumadin), a blood thinner. BotanicLab, the manufacturer of PC SPES, announced a voluntary recall after being confronted with this information, and has since gone out of business.

Others tested four lots of PC SPES and found it to contain small but variable amounts of estrogen in the form of diethylstilbestrol (DES).[75]

The news kept getting worse. A collaborative abstract appeared[76] by researchers in California and the Czech Republic in which the authors analyzed lots of PC SPES manufactured from 1996 to 2001. The researchers found indomethacin and DES contamination of PC SPES, and, in lots after 1999 the researchers found warfarin to be present.

What happened? Was the supplier of herbs in China supplying an adulterated product to BotanicLab? Did the tests for Coumadin actually detect phyto-coumarin, a naturally occurring blood thinner? Did someone decide to spike PC SPES with blood thinner to prevent its side effect of blood clots? Was PC SPES sabotaged? One can only speculate.

Suddenly, men who were holding their cancer at bay with PC SPES had to find other options.

Meanwhile, the original researcher who developed PC SPES, Dr. Sophie Chen, is working with patient organizations and the federal government to bring back PC SPES. Dr. Chen says that, "I stand by the scientific integrity and health benefit of PC SPES on prostate cancer."

---

[75] Small, Eric J: Editorial Comment. UROLOGY 60 (3) 2002:59-60.

[76] Sovak M, Seligson AL, Konas M, Hajduch M, Dolezal M, Machala M, Nagourney R: PC SPES In Prostate Cancer: an Herbal Mixture Currently Containing Warfarin and Previously Diethylstilbestrol and Indomethacin. *Proceedings of the American Association of Cancer Research* 43:LB152, 2002 (abstr), San Francisco, CA April 6-10.

When I Get Prostate Cancer

When I get prostate cancer, I want my tumor cells to be placed inside mice, and if they grow, I want tests done with PC SPES, hormone blocking agents, estrogen, other herbs, and chemotherapeutic agents.

Where can I get this done? Nowhere that I know of. And that's what's wrong with cancer treatment today. Currently, we try to come up with a treatment that works for everyone. There should be more emphasis on coming up with treatments that work for one person, such as individualized chemotherapy and prostate cancer vaccines.

Apparently, there are natural substances in PC SPES that kill prostate cancer. We need to identify and study them. We need to examine the entire Chinese way of medicine where several agents are given, which are thought to act synergistically, while in Western Medicine, typically one medicine is used.

We need to be studying low dose estrogen and the components of PC SPES. There is so much more that could be done for the individual with prostate cancer than is being done!

Bringing Back PC SPES

Dr. Fulton Saier, an obstetrician-gynecologist, told his primary care physician, "I feel excellent. I feel just as good as when I was a teenager," when he went in for a general physical at age fifty-six.

It shocked him when his PSA level was reported to be sky high, at 52 ug/L (normal being 0 to 4). Fulton's PSA had been normal at less than 1.0 only four years earlier.

Fulton's biopsy in October 1999 revealed that 90 percent of the tissue from the left lobe of the prostate was cancerous and 10 percent from the right lobe was cancerous. His Gleason score was 8 to 9. A computerized tomography (CT) scan revealed swelling in the area of the seminal vesicles, suggesting spread of the cancer outside of his prostate. His prognosis was dire.

Fulton presented his diagnosis to his son who, at the time, was obtaining a Masters Degree in Medical Informatics, the science of advancing medicine through information technology.

"I don't like what I'm reading," Fulton's son said, knowing that Fulton's prostate cancer had probably escaped his prostate based on his PSA, Gleason score, and CT scan. "I found this one thing that may be your best shot, Dad," he added.

Fulton's son had found an article about PC SPES and, after Fulton also researched the product; Fulton decided to try PC SPES. Starting November 1, 1999 he took 9 pills per day. Two weeks later, his PSA was 6.0. Two weeks later it was 1.5. Eight weeks later it was non-detectable.

Fulton's prostate decreased in size by 90 percent after PC SPES according to his ultrasound test and according to his doctor's digital rectal examination of Fulton's prostate.

Side Effects per Fulton Saier

"I've had some breast tenderness and some breast enlargement that I do not think is noticeable," the thin Dr. Fulton Saier says. "I've also experienced some decrease in libido, but I can still function."

Bringing Back PC SPES

Like thousands of other men, Fulton's very life may depend on bringing PC SPES back. Fulton is taking the last of his dwindling supply of PC SPES. He has rationed himself to 3 capsules of PC SPES per day and supplements his PC SPES with two pills of a product with similar components called PC PLUS (now called Prostasol).

Several products have sprung up to fill the void left by PC SPES, products such as Prostasol (PC PLUS), PC Care, PC Calm, PC-RES, and Equiguard. But, at this time, none of these other products has the scientific evidence showing they are as effective in placing prostate cancer into remission as PC SPES does.

It is clear that men need PC SPES back, not only for prostate cancer, but because it may be effective against other cancers as well.

Fulton believes that PC SPES saved his life. His only other viable option when he was diagnosed was combined hormone blockade, which would have made him weak and impotent. "I have been on PC SPES since November 1999, and I have led an essentially normal life," Fulton concludes.

Epilogue

Sophie Chen's brother-in-law, the very first PC SPES patient is alive as of March 2003, but like many other men, needs PC SPES to be brought back as quickly as possible.

What You Can Do to Bring PC SPES Back

Today, no manufacturer within the United States has been found who will produce PC SPES. This is a disaster for prostate cancer patients.

Dr. Fulton Saier says, "The National Advisory Counsel for Complementary and Alternative Medicine (NACCAM) to the National Institutes of Health has already voiced strong support for PC SPES by voting (August 26, 2002) to maintain three of their four PC SPES research studies open."

What can you do? Men interested in taking a PC SPES analog, if and when it becomes available, may begin by following the message board at: SurvivingProstateCancerWithoutSurgery.org.

In addition, people interested in assisting NAPC's efforts should write their Congresspersons in Washington, DC. Men with prostate cancer should make them aware of their own health situation and strong desire to have a clean PC SPES analog available for themselves and other men with prostate cancer.

I went to www.Senate.gov and e-mailed my senators, Richard Durbin and Peter Fitzgerald about bringing back PC SPES. Then I went to www.House.gov and wrote my representative, Lane Evans. I hope you will write your senators and representative as well. It is a tragedy that PC SPES, which may be the most effective and safest prostate cancer treatment today, is not available.

Ninety-two studies about PC SPES are currently listed at the National Library of Medicine. Potential users of PC SPES should definitely read these two:

1. de la Taille A, Buttyan R, Hayek O, Bagiella E, Shabsigh A, Burchardt M, Burchardt T, Chopin DK, Katz AE.: Herbal therapy PC-SPES: in vitro effects and evaluation of its efficacy in 69 patients with prostate cancer. *Journal of Urology.* 2000 Oct;164(4):1229-34.

2. Small EJ, Frohlich MW, Bok R, Shinohara K, Grossfeld G, Rozenblat Z, Kelly WK, Corry M, Reese DM.: Prospective trial of the herbal supplement PC-SPES in patients with progressive prostate cancer. *Journal of Clinical Oncology.* 2000 Nov 1;18(21):3595-603.

Estrogen

What some men have learned from the PC SPES fiasco is that taking estrogen, especially with herbal medications may control their prostate cancer.

Many men started taking low-dose estrogen when PC SPES went off the market. In fact, around the world, diethylstilbestrol (one form of estrogen) is a common prostate cancer treatment because it's cheap.

One of the biggest questions is what dose of estrogen is low enough and safe enough to take, while still being effective.

The old doses of estrogen for prostate cancer were 1 to 3 mg per day. Taking doses like 5 mg per day is like being castrated, because it sends your testosterone levels so low, but that dose was stopped because it was too dangerous. It was lowered to 1 to 3 mg per day, but estrogen at that dose is still dangerous; I suspect that it was one of those higher doses that killed my Uncle Steve.

Estrogen has many side effects. Since it suppresses testosterone, you get all the side effects that go with that, including breast enlargement, decreased libido and so on. In addition, in men, estrogen is notorious for causing heart attacks, strokes, and blood clots to the lungs. Estrogen may have to be avoided, or monitored very carefully, in all men who have, or are at risk for, heart disease.

What's interesting is that, besides the suppression of testosterone mechanism for slowing down prostate cancer, some postulate that estrogen has a direct toxic effect on prostate cancer.

Estrogen is also paradoxical, because men who have higher estrogen levels are supposed to be more likely to get prostate cancer. Allegedly, that is why men who eat a high fat diet are more likely to get prostate cancer.

I am following, as an observer only, a group of men on the Internet, who on their own, are taking PC-Plus (now called Prostasol), combined with Honvan, a form of estrogen. Someday, I hope that a randomized controlled trial will be done on this combination therapy. Some of these men have seen spectacular successes in terms of their PSA levels.

The major problem with estrogen is that it can result in blood clots. Taking a small amount of oral blood thinner, usually warfarin (Coumadin), mitigates the problem. These medicines, estrogen and warfarin should be taken under the direction of an expert physician.

There are also those who are adding estrogen and warfarin to the testicle blockers, Lupron or Zoladex. The one thing that is certain is that more studies are needed in this area.

Although this book is almost entirely about localized prostate cancer, men should be aware of an article on advanced prostate cancer about men with positive lymph nodes but without metastases. The author, W. Reid Pitts, MD, FACS, concludes that the immediate use of estrogen (DES 1 mg/day) is the only treatment shown to slow prostate cancer and provide a survival benefit.[77]

---

[77] Pitts WR Jr.: The clinical rationale for immediate androgen deprivation without estrogen deprivation. *Clin Prostate Cancer*. 2003 Sep;2(2):127-8.

Cryoablation of the Prostate

57-year-old Ed Gross suffered an episode of severe pain and urinary frequency in August of 1998. He made the obligatory trip to the urologist where he heard the snapping on of a latex glove and felt the cold chill of K-Y jelly on his behind. He suffered what he thought was surely the rectal exam of a lifetime. He was given a diagnosis of prostatitis and the urologist prescribed antibiotics.

Ed's PSA after a month of antibiotic treatment was 9.4. His PSA the year before had been 2.4. After another three-week program of antibiotics his PSA dropped to 5.2. It stayed in that range until January 1999 when it went to 6.8.

Ed's urologist had previously mentioned the possibility of a prostate biopsy, and with this latest rise in Ed's PSA level he said, "We need to do it now." Ed agreed; he was a zombie who would agree to anything because the big "C" had been looming in the background all this time. The day of the biopsy he took an enema and swallowed an antibiotic per the urologist's instructions. He told himself that he would be strong and calm for the biopsy, but it didn't work out that way. Halfway through the procedure and three snaps of the biopsy gun, Ed began to experience sweating, faintness, and nausea. The urologist offered to stop, but Ed willed himself to get it over with. He certainly didn't want to stop, only to go through the same ordeal all over again. After it was done it took another ten minutes for Ed to calm down and feel better.

A week later he got the call. "Sorry to tell you this, Ed, but one of the biopsies was malignant. You need to come in so we can go over it in more detail."

"Of course," Ed answered trying to stay steady, but he was numb. His mother was just getting over surgery for breast cancer and now this. There was no way he could tell her.

Ed's future became clouded by doom. Because things had been going so well—he was so happy—a feeling overcame him that whatever was wrong, it was going to turn out to be the worst.

Ed's urologist informed him that his malignancy only showed up in one sample—only one core out of six was positive for cancer. He told Ed that his Gleason score was six and that based on his rectal exam he was stage T2 (the urologist thought he could feel a nodule on the prostate). A second pathologist confirmed that Ed's Gleason score was six.

The urologist went into his pitch mode for the radical prostatectomy. He told Ed that although only one core out of six was positive he could not rule cancer out in other areas. The biopsy just may not have hit it. This supported his recommendation for the radical prostatectomy, and besides, even though he felt the cancer was confined to the prostate, during surgery he would sample some lymph nodes. He informed Ed that the radical prostatectomy was the best solution and a cure for his cancer. Ed asked about radiation and seed implants and the urologist admitted that if he went to see a radiation oncologist that they would recommend radiation therapy. Ed seriously considered radiation seed implants for a time, but Ed knew a man who had seeds and he was experiencing urinary irritation. Ed asked about cryoablation. Ed's urologist downplayed it as having too little data.

Ed, who works as the administrator of a cancer surgery unit, read about the sexual dysfunction, urinary incontinence, and urethral strictures (scarring and narrowing of the urethra) caused by the radical prostatectomy. He felt that there had to be a better way. The probability of never having normal sex again was unacceptable. Ed was a sexually active man and couldn't bear the thought of being made impotent. Ed's friend had a radical prostatectomy at age 49 and he was impotent and incontinent.

But Ed's urologist said there were remedies for impotence. Hell, even Bob Dole was telling Ed on TV that there was sex after the radical prostatectomy. But Ed did not find injections into his penis, penile implants, or other sexual aids very appealing. He shuddered at the thought of what his sex life would be like, and expected that his Golden Years would be single and sexless if he underwent a radical prostatectomy. In addition, Ed discovered, much to his surprise, that the studies on the radical prostatectomy were often more propaganda than science. He read about many experts who thought so too. Some even thought that the radical prostatectomy had never cured anyone.

"How could this be?" Ed wondered. He knew that surgery was done all the time. He also knew that virtually every man at the local prostate support group that had surgery was impotent. Worse, the support group was not very supportive about other options.

In April 1999, Ed went for a second opinion at MD Anderson Cancer Center in Houston. He found out that they had been doing cryoablation but had stopped because Medicare wouldn't pay for it. However, Medicare had approved the procedure in February 1999, so MD Anderson was about to begin doing it again. But Ed was worried that the doctors at MD Anderson now lacked experience in the latest techniques of cryoablation. He wanted an experienced physician. He went back to the Internet and began to look very hard at cryoablation, a procedure by which prostate cancer is literally frozen.

History

Cryo means cold. Cryoablation, cryosurgery, and cryotherapy are all terms for freezing prostate cancer.

Cryoblation is done by inserting probes through the skin between the scrotum and anus (the perineum) and into the prostate. Cooling substances circulate through the tip of the probes and freeze prostate cancer. Beforehand, a warming catheter is placed into the urethra to protect it from freezing.

Cryoablation has been around for a long time. As far back as the 1960s cryoablation compared favorably with the radical prostatectomy and radiation therapy for prostate cancer in terms of survival. In fact, a study of 229 cases of cryoablation done between 1969 and 1976 demonstrated experience with cryoablation predating the modern version of the radical prostatectomy.[78] The same study verified comparable survival between cryoablation and the radical prostatectomy as they were both performed at that time.

The problem with cryoablation in the 1960s and 70s was controlling the complications. The most ominous of which were rectal fistulas. A rectal fistula is when a hole develops between the urethra and the rectum. It's a disaster that leads to constant urinary infections. Today, the problem of rectal fistulas has virtually been eliminated.

Radiologist Gary Onik performed the first modern version of cryoablation of the prostate in 1990. His first patient had a high Gleason score of 8, and went for 13 years without metastatic disease after cryoablation. Dr. Onik revolutionized cryoablation by demonstrating—for the first time—that by watching with transrectal ultrasound, a radiologist could see the part of the prostate that was being frozen.

Onik, who is now Director of Surgical Imaging at the Center for the Advancement of Surgery and Celebration of Health continues to do cryoablation today, incorporating new techniques that he has developed. Others, such as radiologists Fred Lee and Duke Bahn, and urologists Jeffrey Cohen and Israel Barkin have also been pioneers in cryoablation.

---

[78] Bonney WW, Fallon B, Gerber WL, Hawtrey CE, Loening SA, Narayana AS, Platz CE, Rose EF, Sall JC, Schmidt JD, and Culp DA: Cryosurgery in prostate cancer: Survival. UROLOGY. January 1982;19(1):37-42.

One improvement is that today instead of using liquid nitrogen as the cooling agent, argon gas is used. The argon gas allows for smaller probe handles and hoses, which means they can be placed closer together. Argon allows for more rapid freezing and thus improved cancer destruction. Argon also allows for more precise freezing.

In 1994, Dr. Gary Onik invented an additional improvement. He now injects the space between the rectum and prostate with normal saline (salt water) to widen that space. This allows cryoablation to be done more completely without fear of injuring the rectum. Since instituting this technique, Dr. Onik has only seen three recurrences out of 270 patients, and those three were simply retreated with cryoablation.[79]

Ed

For Ed, cryoablation was tempting. By all accounts, he had a small pea-sized or smaller cancer in the right side of his prostate. It was probably slow-growing. It was probably not highly aggressive. Ed was sick of the word "probably." He couldn't just watch and wait on the basis of "probably."

Ed listed all the advantages of cryoablation. It isn't major surgery. Since only four to six needles are used to insert into the prostate, some men don't even need to take pain medication after cryoablation. Pain was an important consideration after what he went through with the biopsy.

Cryosurgery is over and done with in one day. Tissue that is frozen is reabsorbed. When nerves are frozen their sheaths remains intact, which may allow regeneration to occur and sometimes return of normal function to those nerves. Bleeding is minimal.

Although not important in Ed's case, doctors can freeze tissue far outside of the prostate, getting to cancer

---

[79] Onik Gary, personal communication with the author by email. March 26th 2003.

that would remain behind at a radical prostatectomy. This means that cryoablation can be used on more advanced cancers, freezing tumors that have escaped the prostate's capsule.

Since doctors are watching what they are doing with ultrasound, cryoablation can be more precise than other therapies. No foreign body is left inside the prostate as is done with radiation seed implants. This, and the fact that cryoablation involves less needle sticks, means that men tolerate cryoablation better than radiation seed implants. Radiation, in any of its forms, causes irritation of the bladder and urethra while cryoablation does not cause this kind of irritation. Ed also worried that any form of radiation therapy held a very small risk of causing bladder or rectal cancer five or ten years down the road—a chance he was not willing to take.

Ed felt that a remarkable advantage of cryoablation is that it can be repeated if necessary. A man with prostate cancer can have cryoablation done once. If later, his PSA rises and a new biopsy shows prostate cancer is present again, he can have cryoablation again—no harm no foul, since cryoablation can be redone without significant complications unlike other therapies. He would also still have all the other options available—hormone blockade, radiation therapy, watchful waiting, and even surgery—the thing he was trying to avoid.

Ed particularly liked the fact that cryoablation could be targeted to the cancer. He didn't want to sacrifice his entire prostate and both seminal vesicles as is always done with surgery. It seemed irrational to Ed to take out so much of a man for a pea-sized tumor.

In the old days surgeons used to lop off the entire breast when a women had breast cancer. Today they usually only remove the cancerous lump and a minor amount of surrounding tissue. Cryosurgery, as Dr. Onik and others are doing it, may be the male version of the lumpectomy. Instead of removing the entire prostate, only the cancerous part is ablated, preserving most function.

For Ed, Dr. Onik would go in and freeze only the cancerous right side of his prostate, its neurovascular bundle, and the seminal vesicle on that side. The doctor could leave all the arteries, veins, and nerves important to his sex life on the other side alone. If his PSA went back up cryoablation would be repeated.

A Special Feature

A fascinating paper about cryoablation appeared in 1971.[80] Doctors treated five men with metastatic prostate cancer. After cryoablation (some men's prostates were frozen more than once) all the metastases disappeared in all the patients. It may be that when prostate cancer is frozen it is like vaccinating against it. The process of freezing prostate cancer may release cancer proteins into the circulation, which men's bodies learn to attack. Going back and refreezing the tumor again may be like giving a booster shot, revving up the body's immune system again against the cancer. Doctors are still trying to figure out why, and with what technique, this phenomenon of revving up the immune system with cryoablation may occur.

Two approaches to cryoablation are emerging. One school believes that the entire prostate should be frozen along with the nerve trunks on both sides of the prostate. Some doctors choose this approach because it should be the most likely way of being sure to freeze all the cancer that may be present. But it also results in a high rate of impotence, although, even with total freezing, about 15 to 20 percent of men in this fashion regain potency.

Two radiologists, Duke Bahn, and Fred Lee, at Crittendon Hospital in Rochester, Michigan are representative of the total freezing approach. They may have the most experience with cryoablation in the world as they

---

[80] Ablin RJ, Soanes WA, and Gonder MJ: Prospects for Cryo-Immunotherapy in Cases of Metastasizing Carcinoma of the Prostate. *Cryobiology* 1971;8(3):271-279.

have treated over 725 men. These two physicians are also renowned for their philosophy of patient empowerment and education. Their biopsy proven 5-year cure rate for T1 and T2 (locally confined) cancer is virtually 90 percent, while for T3 and T4 (locally spread) cancers it is 79 percent. The incontinence rate among their patients is only 4.3 percent (wearing diapers or pads), and the majority of that is stress incontinence only.

Dr. Onik uses both approaches depending on the extent of the tumor inside a man, but he believes that the beauty of cryoablation is that it can be targeted to the tumor. One-half of the prostate and its nerve trunks can often be spared. The targeted approach is more likely to save sexual function, and cryosurgery can be repeated if necessary.

Ed's Cryoablation

Ed leans toward the profile of the typical man to undergo cryoablation. The stereotype of the man who chooses cryoablation is that he is college educated or above, owns his own business, is an engineer, has done an incredible amount of research on his own, and is extremely well-informed. Ed was so well-informed he felt like he deserved a medical degree.

Ed met with Dr. Onik, who suggested a more extensive biospy to make certain that the cancer was indeed small and localized. Ed agreed and drove to Orlando, where Dr. Onik mercifully performed the biopsy procedure under general anesthesia. Ed woke up feeling great and ready to drive back to Miami, but that's a no-no after general anesthesia, so he stayed with friends.

"Great news," Dr. Onik reported to Ed one week later. "It's localized only in the right base." He advised Ed that he was a candidate for partial cryoablation, which Ed had hoped for all along, where only part of the right lobe would be frozen.

"Let's do it," Ed said. He felt this was a prostate cancer treatment option that he could live with.

Ed underwent a liquid diet for two days prior to the procedure. The morning of the surgery he arose at 6 a.m. and cleaned out his colon with several enemas—thankfully, no laxatives and explosive diarrhea were needed to prepare for cryoablation. He drove four and one-half hours from Miami to Orlando for the procedure.

At noon Ed was wheeled into the operating room. He was given general anesthesia and went to sleep. A urethral warmer was inserted into his penis and an ultrasound probe was inserted into his rectum. Four probes were passed through the skin of his perineum into his prostate. Dr. Onik injected the space between his prostate and rectum with saline. Cold argon gas was introduced into the probes and the right side of Ed's prostate was frozen and thawed three times along with his right neurovascular bundle and seminal vesicle. The equipment was removed from Ed, a Foley catheter was placed in his bladder, and he was sent to the recovery room.

Ed awoke from anesthesia with pain, but a shot of Demerol quickly ended it. After that he only used Tylenol or his bladder anti-spasm medication. He never had to use any of the stronger pain pills he was prescribed.

Most men go home the same day, but since Ed had driven four and one-half hours to get to the hospital, he went home the next day instead.

Ed wore his urinary catheter and "leg bag" for three weeks. He returned to work after only three days at home. Besides the catheter, the only other discomfort after the surgery was swelling of his scrotum, which took about ten days to subside.

Ed experienced some urinary stinging and burning for a week after the catheter was removed, but then he was back to normal. Ed's PSA level has stabilized since the procedure and Ed is confident that he chose the least harmful way of treating his prostate cancer. Almost two years after the procedure Ed's PSA level is still holding steady between 2.4 and 3.0. Because he had only half his gland frozen, Ed's PSA is not expected to go to zero. Ed will be watching for three PSA rises in row, not for any certain target level of PSA.

Side Effects

Today, cryoablation patients suffer rectal fistula formation only about 0.4 percent of time and usually only if men were irradiated prior to cryoablation. In Dr. Onik's series this complication has been eliminated due to the saline injections between the prostate and rectum. Urethral sloughing and bladder neck contractures can occur, but are rare.

Minor complications include trouble with urination about 10 percent of the time, pelvic pain in about 11 percent of men, scrotal swelling in 17 percent of men, and penile numbness or a tingling sensation in 14 percent. These are usually temporary complications that resolve within three months after cryoablation.

When cryoablation is done on larger cancers, more side effects occur. A 1996 study of 102 men mentioned several complications from cryoablation in men with more extensive disease (often the men had T3 tumors, those that have spread beyond the capsule of the prostate). Many men had to wear a suprapubic urinary catheter for 2 to 55 days because of urinary obstruction. Urinary obstruction occurred in 25 percent of the patients, and this obstruction was often delayed, happening 2 to 3 months after cryoablation. The incontinence rate was 4 percent from cryoablation alone but increased to 15 percent when additional men became incontinent after undergoing a TURP for obstruction. Penile numbness occurred in 10 percent of the men and lasted as long as 10 months before resolving. The impotence rate at one year was 84 percent.

There was a 10 percent rate of rectourethral fistula in men who had already had radiation therapy.[81]

On the upside, the complications mentioned above are being reduced, even in extensive cryoablation procedures, due to saline injections, newly designed urethral warmers, and better temperature monitoring. Despite the complications that sometimes occur with cryoablation, most men are able to resume their normal activities in a matter of weeks.

One almost can't help but cheer for cryoablation. It's less expensive, has fewer side effects, and is certainly a lot less painful than major surgery. Dr. Onik says:

> "I expect that within five years we will see the death of the radical prostatectomy as a treatment for prostate cancer."[82]

Urologist Israel Barkin, who uses every method of treating prostate cancer: radiation, radiation seeds, watchful waiting, cryoablation, and hormone blockade, quit doing the radical prostatectomy in 1992 because so few men want it when they know about all the other options.

After years of struggle by health-care activists, Medicare finally agreed to reimburse for cryoablation in February 1999. Sadly, many feel that cryoablation reimbursement rates have been set too low because of the influence of powerful urologists who do not want competition for their most lucrative surgery.

You should be fighting mad about how urologists have interfered with the advancement of cryoablation. I am. In my view, urologists have inappropriately blocked the progress of cryoablation in order to preserve the right to do radical surgery.

---

[81] Connolly JA, Shinohara K, Presti Jr. JC, and Carroll PR: Should cryosurgery be considered a therapeutic option in localized prostate cancer? *Urologic Clinics of North America*. November 1996;23(4):623-631.

[82] Onik, Gary: telephone conversation with the author on December 9, 1999. Quoted with signed, written permission.

Cryoablation is not the only procedure that urologists may have helped block. Neotonus Incorporated is suing the American Urological Association claiming that the organization is blocking their NeoControl incontinence treatment. A newspaper reported that the suit claims the AUA "classified the technology as experimental because they feared the treatment would lessen the need for surgery and hurt urologists' incomes."[83]

Ed's Outcome

I checked with Ed on August 9, 2004 and his prostate cancer remains in remission. His PSA has held steady at 2.9, which is fine for someone with half a prostate. He hasn't suffered any serious side effects from cryoablation. He has no incontinence at all, even when coughing or straining. The sensation to Ed's penis is fine. Best of all, except for a decreased amount of semen, Ed's sex life is back to normal. Sometimes Ed is so exuberant with his outcome that he can't help but shake his arms in joy and yell, "Yes!" Since Ed's cancer was discovered at age 57, and 5 years later Ed is in remission, Ed appears to have made a great choice.

Cryosurgery to Save other Failed Treatments

Archbishop Desmond Tutu had radiation therapy and then when his cancer returned underwent salvage cryoablation by Dr. H. Clark at Emory University in November 1999.

In 1987, 60-year-old Plato Jones underwent a routine physical before embarking on a cruise. "The doctor said he wanted to talk after I returned. I should have been alarmed, but I wasn't," Plato told me.

---

[83] Megan Woolhouse: Tiny health firm sues 2 Goliaths. *Atlanta Business Chronicle.* Aug. 8, 2004.

Plato is sleek of build. He looks scholarly in his glasses, has a salt and pepper mustache, and alert brown eyes. Most importantly, he is very open about talking about his prostate cancer.

After the cruise, Plato's doctor told him that his prostate was too big. Plato was sent to a urologist who performed a biopsy, which was positive for prostate cancer. Plato couldn't believe it. In his words, he was angry, mad, and upset. The urologist recommended surgery. His wife wanted surgery, but his internist wanted him to talk to a radiation oncologist. "I underwent radiation, and I'm so glad that I did," Plato says today. "I've heard all the stories of the guys who had surgery." Plato underwent external beam radiation 5 days per week for six to seven weeks.

"How did the radiation affect your sexual function?"

"My wife doesn't think it affected sex at all. I think it did a little bit," Plato says.

"What about men who had surgery then?"

"They were dead sexually," Plato replied. (To be fair, both surgery and radiation therapy have improved drastically since 1987.)

Plato did have some diarrhea, which subsided and became tolerable over the years. He also had irritable bladder with urinary frequency, which became better with time.

Plato essentially recovered almost completely, and has traveled all over the world since his treatment. But in 1998, his PSA, which had always hovered around 2.0, went up to 4. By 1999 his PSA was up to 5.0. A CT scan, bone scan, and prostate biopsy were all negative. His PSA went up to 6.0. On May 12, 2000 Plato underwent another prostate biopsy and it was positive for prostate cancer.

On September 25th, 2000 Plato underwent cryoablation by Dr. James K. Bennet in Atlanta. He was under general anesthesia during the procedure.

"They gave me a second belly button," Plato said, as a way of describing the suprapubic catheter that was placed to drain his urine. Plato could urinate through his penis after the procedure, but only in small amounts. The catheter drained the "residual urine" from his bladder.

However, after only 2 days the supra-pubic catheter was removed and Plato was urinating normally again. Plato has been suffering some urinary incontinence since the cryoablation, which he hopes will go away. He has been wearing one maxi-pad per day. He is also doing Kegel exercises. "They work. The damn Kegel exercises actually work," he says clearly pleased.

"Sex now?"

"My risk of impotence is 50/50 after cryo," Plato says, but he adds, "At age 73 I no longer care about sex."

Plato's experience points out an important new role for cryoablation, which is being the salvage therapy after other therapies—surgery or radiation—fail. Only 10 days after Plato's cryoablation he was speaking to me after attending an Us TOO meeting at Emory University. He looked fine, like nothing at all had ever happened.[84]

Complications

Dr. Duke Bahn and Fred Lee of Crittenton Hospital in Rochester Hills, Michigan, and their colleagues, did one of the best papers on the side effect rate of cryoablation. They surveyed the first patients they treated with cryoablation resulting in a study group of 223 men.[85] But remember, unlike what Ed had done, in this study of side effects, the doctors froze the entire prostate and neurovascular bundles on both sides. The results were:

- 9 percent of the continent men before cryo used pads after cryoablation

---

[84] Jones, Plato. Interview with the author. Used with signed, written permission, October 4, 2000.
[85] Badalament RA, Bahn DK, Kim H, Kumar A, Bahn JM, and Lee F: Patient-reported complications after cryoablation therapy for prostate cancer. UROLOGY. 1999:54(2):295-300.

- 85 percent of the potent men became impotent after cryoablation
- A urethra to rectum fistula occurred in one patient
- Urinary obstruction occurred in 10 percent of the men, requiring dilation or transurethral resection of the prostate
- Scrotal swelling occurred in 18 percent
- Penile tingling occurred in 15 percent
- Pelvic pain occurred in 12 percent.

The last three symptoms typically resolved over a three-month period.

Charlie Russ

When Charlie Russ, a flamboyant attorney, came down with prostate cancer, he underwent a radical prostatectomy and the cancer returned. He then underwent radiation therapy and it also failed.

Charlie became a volunteer attorney for PAACT to help men get reimbursed for cryoablation. He battled Medicare, urologists, and the courts to achieve coverage.

Charlie, before he passed away, said, "If I could, I would sue every urologist." Charlie was truly mad at how much urologists were looking out for themselves instead of for patients. His was one of the many stories that made me look hard at current urological practices.

After the death of Charlie Russ, Gregory H. Teuful, Esq. of Schnader, Harrison, Segal, & Lewis LLP, a law firm in Pennsylvania, has been instrumental in helping men get reimbursed for cryoablation by Medicare. He is now contemplating bringing suit against Medicare for setting the fee reimbursement schedule too low. The low rate of reimbursement for cryoablation only serves to delay research into this promising new procedure.

Once again, one cannot help but cheer for cryoablation; it has had to overcome so many obstacles.

Results

The results that are emerging for cryoablation done by the best people are truly amazing. In a study of 590 consecutive men treated with cryoablation for localized or locally advanced prostate cancer, only 13 percent of men had biopsies positive for prostate cancer after treatment, and those men were simply treated again.[86]

---

[86] Bahn DK, Lee F, Badalament R, Kumar A, Greski J, and Chernick M: Targeted Cryoablation of the Prostate: 7-Year Outcomes in the Primary Treatment of Prostate Cancer. Abstract to appear in a supplement to UROLOGY. 2002.

Hormone Blockade for prostate cancer

Hormone blockade has increased survival for prostate cancer patients according to one randomized controlled trial.[87] Which is why, after watchful waiting, active non-invasive therapy, PC SPES, perhaps low dose estrogen, and some kind of local therapy such as cryoablation or radiation, I would turn to hormone blockade next. The reason I would not turn to hormone blockade before those other things for localized prostate cancer is quality of life. Although, I would consider moving hormone blockade higher on my list depending on the type and size of prostate cancer that I had, or if another randomized controlled study confirmed the results of the first study. I might also take hormone-blockade while researching what else to do. Preventing metastases is very important in prostate cancer.

In 1966, Dr. Charles Brenton Huggins won the Nobel Prize in medicine for discovering that testosterone influenced prostate cancer. His work led doctors to the rather horrific practice of castrating men with advanced prostate cancer. However, for some men it seemed worth it, as sometimes, dramatic remissions would result.

Soon, it was found that instead of castration, estrogen—sort of the opposite of testosterone—could be given for advanced prostate cancer. However, at the doses being given to men back then, there were side effects of blood clotting and heart attacks, and estrogen treatment for

---

[87] Labrie F, Candas B, Dupont A, Cusan L, Gomez JL, Suburu RE, Diamond P, Levesque J, Belanger A: Screening decreases prostate cancer death: first analysis of the 1988 Quebec prospective randomized controlled trial. *Prostate.* 1999 Feb 1;38(2):83-91.

prostate cancer fell out of favor. Estrogen caused as many deaths as it prevented.

For a while, castration, gruesome as it was, remained cheap and unbeatable as a treatment.

Lloyd Ney

In 1983, doctors diagnosed Lloyd Ney Sr. with advanced prostate cancer. His cancer had escaped his prostate and had penetrated into surrounding tissues (Stage T3). Ney underwent 30 external beam radiation treatments to his prostate, but afterwards, x-rays revealed that his cancer had spread to his bones (Stage T4). "You have six months to live," his urologist reportedly told him.

Only 65, Lloyd Ney, Sr., PhD, found his death sentence unacceptable. He researched prostate cancer on his own and discovered a therapy called hormone blockade. He flew to Quebec City, Canada, and underwent hormone blockade under the supervision of Fernand Labrie, MD, PhD, one of its pioneers.

Outraged that his doctors didn't even tell him about hormone blockade, Lloyd Ney founded the nonprofit group, Patient Advocates for Advanced Cancer Treatments (PAACT). PAACT is alleged to be the oldest prostate cancer support group in existence, and Lloyd Ney deserves much of the credit for bringing hormone blockade therapy to the United States. Dr. Ney and PAACT changed the history of prostate cancer, and PAACT continues to be an excellent resource for men.

Ney would live for *14 more years* after his death sentence, all the while on hormone blockade, until he died at age 79 in 1998. Ney would actually die of repeat urinary tract infections from radiation damage to his bladder. He regretted ever having radiation and believed that hormone blockade would have been sufficient for him.

PAACT makes every attempt to provide up-to-date information on hormone blockade. PAACT is associated with the Prostate Cancer Oncology Group (PCOG), which vigilantly surveys the medical literature to provide the best information to patients.

Lloyd Ney once wrote that combination hormone blockade " . . . is the first and mandatory treatment regardless of the initial stage of the disease."[88]

Lloyd Ney may have been right, and while we wait for hard scientific proof, I recommend that you contact PAACT for their latest information on hormone blockade therapy.

---

[88] Ney, Lloyd: PAACT. Detection, Diagnosis, Evaluation, and Treatment of Prostate Cancer. Revised 1997.

Hormone Blockade Details

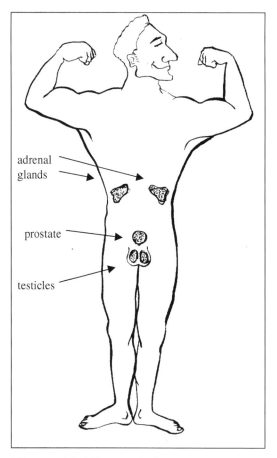

Figure 14. The male hormones are produced by three organs, the adrenal glands, the prostate, and the testicles. (Artist: Jun Macam)

Introduction

The testicles, the adrenal glands, and the prostate all produce male hormones. The testicles produce the largest amount, the adrenal glands a smaller percentage, and the prostate produces the least amount.

Each of these three organs produces different hormones. The testicles produce testosterone, the adrenal glands secrete several male hormones known collectively as the "adrenal androgens," and the prostate produces dihydrotestosterone (DHT).

One strategy to fight prostate cancer is to block the male hormones. We call such treatment single hormone blockade, double hormone blockade, or triple hormone blockade, depending on how many of the three organs, 1) the testicles, 2) adrenal glands, or 3) the prostate, are blocked.

Today, the old "surgical castration" with a scalpel (orchiectomy) is being replaced by medications that produce "chemical castration." Medications can be stopped, while surgical castration cannot be reversed. Thus, utilizing medications provides more flexibility. It's also no secret that men usually don't want to be castrated.

The names of the hormone blocking medications are difficult. Lupron (leuprolide) and Zoladex (goserelin) block testosterone production by the testicles; they are testicle-blockers. Medications that block the adrenal glands include Eulexin (flutamide), Casodex (biclutamide), and Nilandron (nilutimide); they are "adrenal-blockers."

Medications that work at the level of the prostate to block its production of hormones include Proscar (finasteride), and the herb saw palmetto (*Serenoa repens*) (although the mechanism of saw palmetto is not fully understood); these are the "prostate-blockers."

Blocking the Testicles

The testicle-blockers, Lupron (leuprolide) and Zoladex (goserelin), work indirectly. They affect the pituitary gland in the brain, which in turn affects the testicles. It is easiest simply to think as these drugs as "testicle-blockers" despite the convoluted way in which they work. These two drugs are replacing surgical castration. Blocking testosterone by using these drugs or by castration is called "single hormone blockade."

Lupron and Zoladex may be equally effective, but there are differences between the two in both their administration and their side effects. Lupron is a liquid that is injected into muscle, such as the buttock. Zoladex is a pellet that is implanted beneath the skin of the upper stomach area with a fairly large needle. Many men require local anesthesia of the skin before receiving an injection of a Zoladex pellet.

Because the testicle-blockers imitate testosterone before they block it, they produce an initial surge in testosterone, called the "flare reaction." This flare occurs as these agents first settle in to work. This initial surge in testosterone can cause prostate cancer to enlarge with dire consequences. For example, a man who has prostate cancer in his spine could experience a sudden rapid growth of cancer, compressing his spinal cord, causing paralysis with bowel and bladder incontinence. Similarly, a testosterone flare induced by a testicle-blocker can cause prostate cancer to suddenly grow large enough to interfere with the kidneys or induce it to pinch a nerve.

To prevent the flare reaction, men are almost always started on adrenal-blockers prior to being medicated with testicle-blockers. By blocking the adrenal hormones first, the flare reaction seldom occurs.

The testicle-blockers, Lupron and Zoladex, have serious side effects. They are sexually devastating because they stop testosterone from working. Being on a testicle-blocker can cause your testicles to shrink to the size of peanuts and your penis to shrink nearly as small as it was before puberty set in. Both drugs generally cause impotence and loss of sexual desire.

"My husband's once impressive genitals are no bigger than a 12-year-old's now," to paraphrase what one wife revealed to me about the effects of hormone blockade.

The testicle-blockers also cause fatigue, hot flashes, breast swelling, and nipple tenderness. Men are sometimes advised to undergo breast irradiation to prevent breast enlargement prior to undergoing these medications.

Testicle-blockers should not be taken without a full understanding of their side effects. Some men recover very well from the testicle-blockers. In others their testosterone levels only slowly recover or don't recover at all. For some men, permanent problems with hot flashes and potency can persist after being on these medications.

Blocking the Adrenal Glands

The medications Eulexin (flutamide), Casodex (biclutamide), and Nilandron (nilutamide) block the production of male hormones by the adrenal glands. Thus, these three drugs are "adrenal-blockers."

Eulexin (flutamide) was the first adrenal-blocker to be approved by the FDA, so doctors have the most experience with it. Eulexin is a pill that must be taken on an exact eight-hour schedule, but having to take it frequently also means it is eliminated quickly from your system if you need to be taken off the drug. Casodex (biclutamide) and Nilandron (nilutamide) are pills that need to be taken only once a day, but this also means that they take longer to get out of your system.

Other important differences are emerging between these drugs as studies are being completed and ongoing studies should determine which drug is best for each type of prostate cancer.

What are the adrenal hormones that these drugs are blocking? They are a group of male androgens with long, technical names such as androstenedione and dehydroepiandrosterone (DHEA). The adrenal-blockers can cause liver toxicity, diarrhea, hot flashes, breast pain, weakness, anemia, and other side effects.

Blocking the Prostate

The prostate converts testosterone into a more powerful hormone called dihydrotestosterone (DHT). DHT is thought to be a potent initiator of prostate growth, and probably of prostate cancer growth as well. The enzyme that converts testosterone into DHT is called 5 alpha-reductase. Proscar (finasteride) inhibits this enzyme.

Proscar was the first medication developed for the treatment of benign prostatic hyperplasia (BPH), but it also appears to prevent prostate cancer. In fact, in the "Prostate Cancer Prevention Trial," 18,000 men were randomized to receive either finasteride (Proscar) or placebo. Digital rectal exams and PSA tests were done yearly. The men underwent prostate biopsies at the end of the study. The study found that finasteride decreased the risk of prostate cancer by 25 percent in men over age 55, with normal digital rectal exams and PSAs below 0.3 ng/ml. The men also benefited from improved urination. However, the men suffered some sexual side effects, and in those men who got prostate cancer despite the drug, the cancer tended to have higher Gleason scores. So, less cancer occurred, but the cancer that did occur was worse.

Triple Hormone Blockade

Some physicians are using Proscar (finasteride) as part of combined hormone blockade. It is usually the third medication in such protocols, after a testicle-blocker and an adrenal-blocker.

When the prostate-blocker, Proscar, is added, such protocols are called triple hormone blockade. In triple hormone blockade, the male hormones are being blocked at the testicles, adrenal glands, and the prostate.

Proscar, you may remember, blocks the prostate from converting testosterone into dihydrotestosterone (DHT).

Proscar may also have some innate anti-cancer activity that is just beginning to be understood.

Proscar may interfere with the use of PSA as a cancer test, and thus it is often recommended that men get a baseline PSA before beginning Proscar.

Saw palmetto (*Serenoa repens*) is an herbal preparation that some sources claim works the same way Proscar does. It is also alleged that saw palmetto has anti-inflammatory properties and relaxes urinary smooth muscle. Saw palmetto has been widely used as an over-the-counter treatment for prostatitis and BPH, and it may play a role in slowing down or preventing prostate cancer.

Since these two medications, Proscar and saw palmetto, block hormone production by the prostate, we will refer to them as "prostate-blockers."

Type of medication	Name of medicines
testicle-blockers	Lupron (leuprolide)
	Zoladex (goserelin)
adrenal-blockers	Eulexin (flutamide)
	Casodex (biclutamide)
	Nilandron (nilutamide)
prostate-blockers	Proscar (finasteride)
	saw palmetto (*Serenoa repens*)

Terminology

The terminology is confusing because hormone blockade goes by many names. In studies, it is sometimes hard to tell if the authors are talking about blocking one organ or all three organs. I advocate spelling out single, double, or triple hormone blockade in order to lessen the confusion. And although I prefer the term blockade, other physicians may refer to hormone blocking regimens by any of the following terms:

- Combined hormone blockade (CHB, when more than one organ is being blocked)
- Single hormone blockade (just an LHRH analog is used)
- Double hormone blockade (an LHRH analog and an antiandrogen)
- Triple hormone blockade (an LHRH analog, antiandrogen, and 5 alpha-reductase inhibitor)
- Hormonal ablation therapy (HAT)
- Combined hormone therapy (CHT)
- Total androgen blockade (TAB)
- Androgen deprivation therapy (ADT)
- Intermittent hormone blockade (IHB)
- Complete hormone therapy (CHT)
- Endocrine combination therapy (ECT)
- Hormone deprivation therapy
- Hormone ablation therapy.

Effectiveness

Hormone blockade can be astonishingly effective. Typically, at least 85 percent of men with prostate cancer respond to hormone blockade therapy. Indeed, there are cases where hormone blockade therapy was given before surgery, then after surgery, all evidence of prostate cancer had disappeared when the removed prostate was examined under a microscope.

It sounds too good to be true, and it apparently is, as giving blockade before surgery has not been proven to increase survival at the time of this writing.

The problem with hormone blockade is that prostate cancer may develop resistance to it in many men. The initial enthusiasm for hormone blockade was sky high, but early controlled studies were unable to show that hormone blockade increased survival, only later studies started to show some benefit.

In addition, although usually reversible, the side effects of decreased libido, shrinkage of the genitals, breast development, gastrointestinal trouble, and hot flashes can be hard to tolerate. Such side effects definitely decrease the quality of life. Still, because hormone blockade is at least temporarily effective it is standard therapy for men with *metastatic* prostate cancer. And by using hormone blockade in new fashions and different combinations, some doctors believe they are seeing increases in survival.

Dr. Fernand Labrie

Dr. Fernand Labrie, a physician and endocrinologist, and his colleagues invented medical castration using a testicle-blocker (LHRH agonist). Their first patient was reported in the medical literature in 1980.

Another of Dr. Labrie's ideas was to block the testicles and the adrenal glands simultaneously. Dr. Labrie and his colleagues first did this in 1982. The idea quickly caught on. Today, many men are placed on a testicle-blocker and an adrenal-blocker simultaneously.

The results of double hormone blockade have been encouraging. Studies have shown an average increase in average overall survival of three to six months compared to castration alone. If only men are considered who don't die of some other cause than prostate cancer during the treatment period, the gain is usually six to 12 additional months of life.

Readers may be shocked to realize that, on average, men don't benefit more from treating prostate cancer. This is one of the "dirty secrets" about prostate cancer no one talks about. One decision analysis showed that treating prostate cancer resulted in an average loss of 3.5 months of quality-adjusted life.[89] Another decision analysis found that treating prostate cancer resulted in an average loss of

---

[89] Mold JW, Holtgrave DR, Bisonni RS, Marley DS, Wright RA, Spann SJ: The evaluation and treatment of men with asymptomatic prostate nodules in primary care: a decision analysis. *Journal of Family Practice.* 1992;34(5):561-568.

quality-adjusted life of 1.8 to 9.5 days.[90] The common treatments in the two studies just mentioned were radical prostatectomy and radiation therapy, so by contrast, hormone blockade may look very good to you, depending on how you feel about the quality of life while on hormone blockade.

Hormone Blockade Before Symptoms Occur

Doctors have started asking, why wait for symptoms to occur? Why wait for urinary trouble to develop or for metastases to cause bone pain? Why not give hormone blockade earlier? This in fact is the dramatic question emerging today. How and when do we use hormone blockade? Some studies show that in men with metastatic disease, the fewer the metastases, the better the life-prolonging effects of hormone blockade. So even if the patient has no bone pain from his metastases, it may be that starting blockade immediately will allow him to live longer. There is even a trend in localized prostate cancer to initiate hormone blockade immediately.

More and more, men choose to begin double hormone blockade immediately, and feel that this gives them the time to study all the other options available. After being on hormone blockade and studying the issues, men can go on to have some sort of local therapy done such as a form of radiation, cryoablation, or a radical prostatectomy, or they can continue on hormone blockade as their only therapy.

It's become clear that small localized prostate cancer tumors are much more sensitive to hormone blockade than large tumors that have metastasized. That's why many doctors are considering treating men with prostate cancer immediately upon diagnosis, even men with small, localized cancers.

---

[90] Krahn MD, Mahoney JE, Eckman MH, Trachtenberg J, Pauker SG, Detsky AS: Screening for prostate cancer: a decision analytic view. JAMA. 1994;272:773-780.

Why Does Hormone Blockade Sometimes Fail?

One theory about why hormone blockade eventually fails in many men is that all prostate cancer cells are hormone sensitive in the beginning, and when the male hormones are blocked all prostate cancer cells stop growing. Then, a certain number of cancer cells become independent of male hormones and start growing again. Hormone-independent prostate cancer takes over. Thus, over time, hormone blockade therapy, while initially successful, can fail.

It may also be that prostate cancer is a mixture of hormone-sensitive and hormone-independent cells from the very beginning, and that when the hormone-sensitive cells are shut down by hormone blockade the hormone-independent cells simply take over. A third theory is that prostate cancer adapts to the lack of male hormones by creating more hormone receptors on every cell, becoming so sensitive that even the most minute amount of unblocked hormone can cause the cancer to start growing again.

It's also possible that when the male hormones are blocked, some other substance takes over and drives prostate cancer to grow.

The size of the prostate cancer at diagnosis may make a difference. Small cancers seem to contain all similar cells; all of them sensitive to hormone blockade. Larger cancers have already undergone a lot of change, because as prostate cancer grows it loses its differentiation (becomes bizarrely shaped) and higher Gleason scores are produced. It may be that after these changes hormone blockade simply can't be as effective. This is one of the arguments for starting hormone blockade immediately even with small prostate cancers. Researchers are wondering if doing so would prevent hormone resistance from developing.

Sadly, physicians are still grappling with how to use hormone blockade to the best advantage.

How Should Hormone Blockade be Used?

Traditionally, once hormone blockade has been given it is continued for life. And the studies that have suggested increased survival have been in men who stayed on hormone blockade for five years or more. There are still many questions.

Should single, double, or triple hormone blockade therapy be used? Should hormone blockade be started as soon as prostate cancer is diagnosed, causing serious side effects, or should treatment be held off until the prostate cancer warrants it? Should hormone blockade be given continuously or should it be given intermittently? These are just a few of the many questions that need to be answered.

Some experts think that no matter how well male hormones are blocked, prostate cancer will eventually overcome the blockade. Others believe that double hormone blockade or triple hormone blockade followed by Proscar (finasteride) maintenance (where after a suitable period of triple hormone blockade, the man stops everything but Proscar) can put men into remission for life.

Is Hormone Blockade Better than Surgical Castration?

One of the first questions that needed to be answered with the advent of drugs that were able to cause chemical castration was whether these drugs were a better form of treatment than surgical castration.

A major problem with surgical castration is emotional despair. It is also irreversible. If you have difficult side effects such as hot flashes, you may come to regret having had your testicles removed as a prostate cancer treatment. Aside from the impotence that occurs after castration, the hot flashes, tiredness, and mental dysfunction that may occur and are often disabling. Many men experience problems of concentration so severe that they many not be able to work.[91] Unlike surgical castration, medical castration by hormone blockade can be stopped. You can change your mind or experiment with different doses and medications if problems occur.

"I would never have been castrated if I knew then what I know now," to paraphrase what several men have revealed to me.

Men prefer medical castration because if the side effects of testosterone blockade are horrible, they have more options with drugs. Sadly, surgical removal of the testicles is forever. In addition, if the wonder cure for prostate cancer is discovered tomorrow, it would be a tragedy to have been surgically castrated.

Should Hormone Blockade be Given Before Radiation Seed Implants?

There is also a great deal of debate about whether hormone blockade of some sort should be used prior to radiation seed implants. In theory, such a protocol could kill off any prostate cancer cells that were outside of the prostate, leaving the radioactive seeds to destroy the primary tumor.

This approach is already being used. One of the side benefits is that hormone blockade shrinks the prostate, making the procedure less technically difficult because the physician is working with a smaller prostate.

The theoretical harm is that the hormone blockade won't kill off all the prostate cancer and the cancer that returns will be more aggressive than the original. And the side effects of hormone blockade are significant so men really need to know what works and what doesn't.

There is considerable controversy over how long a patient should be on hormone blockade before seeds are

---

[91] Newling DWW: The palliative therapy of advance prostate cancer, with particular reference to the results of recent European clinical trials. *British Journal of Urology.* 1997;79(suppl 1):72-81.

implanted. Should it be three months, nine months, or a year or more? And should single, double, or triple hormone blockade be used?

Double Hormone Blockade Before Surgery

Several studies have shown that if a testicle-blocker combined with an adrenal-blocker is given for three months prior to a radical prostatectomy, there will be a decrease in the incidence of prostate cancer found to have penetrated the prostate's capsule and of positive surgical margins.[92] Although this sounds marvelous, there is a great deal of controversy about whether such treatment translates to an increase in survival. So far, this technique does not seem to prolong survival. It will take years for this issue to be sorted out.

---

[92] Vaillancourt L, Tetu B, Fradet Y, Dupont A, Gomez J, Cusan L, Suburu ER, Diamond P, Candas B, Labrie F: Effect of Neoadjuvant Endocrine Therapy (Combined Androgen Blockade) on Normal Prostate and Prostatic Carcinoma: a randomized study. *American Journal of Surgical Pathology*. 1996;20(1):86-93.

Intermittent Hormone Blockade and Bud Irish

On April 9, 1945, Aarol "Bud" Irish of Hemlock, Michigan lay next to a fellow soldier who had just been machine-gunned to death by German soldiers. Bud and his friend had been on a reconnaissance mission for the 102nd Mechanized Calvary Unit and the 701st Tank Battalion, one of dozens of missions they had done during World War II, but this one went badly. A German SS officer who emptied his gun into their area killed another of Bud's buddies lying beside him, but every bullet miraculously missed Bud. As the Germans approached, Bud played dead, and was slammed over the head with a gun butt, but he continued his ruse and thus Bud survived the SS troopers. Four of his buddies were killed, but the mission probably saved 1,000 men.

Later, Bud ran a gauntlet of bullets to escape to safety. He found an ambulance and went back to rescue three other men, for which he would be awarded the Silver Star.

Forty-five years later in Saginaw, Michigan, in September 1989, at age 68, the day before Bud was to leave for Holland to reunite with other war veterans, he couldn't urinate. He went to the hospital and was catheterized, his bladder releasing two liters of pent up urine. In December 1989, his first PSA level was 76 and a prostate biopsy later that month revealed cancer. He was advised to have surgery or radiation right away. Instead, Bud went to Venice, Florida, for vacation and to think.

While in Florida, he hooked up with Sarasota urologist Willet Whitmore III. Dr. Whitmore determined that Bud's prostate was enlarged, 85 grams in size, PSA 79, and that he was stage T3 and possibly stage T4 (the cancer had already escaped his prostate. Whitmore started Bud on double hormone blockade with shots of the testicle-blocker Lupron and pills of the adrenal-blocker Eulexin. Within four months, Bud's PSA was virtually undetectable and his prostate was normal in size again. Bud also noted that he could urinate well again.

After eight months, Bud did something that may change prostate cancer history. Bud took himself off both Lupron and Eulexin for a year. Bud, the father of five sons and five daughters, felt that men needed to know what happened if you stopped the medications. Dr. Whitmore told him that he was either going to be a "damn fool or had better be pretty lucky." Bud felt he had been living on borrowed time since 1945 anyway, and was determined to see what happened.

He went off both medications, and after some time his PSA went back up to 13.5. Bud went back on double hormone blockade. In three months his PSA dropped to 1.1. Bud stopped the Eulexin after reading about the possible long-term side effects of the drug, and stayed on Lupron alone for 11 months. He stopped the Lupron also and was off both drugs for seven months before his PSA went up to 7.3. Bud has been going on and off hormone blockade like this for over a decade.

To my knowledge, Bud Irish, who literally did it himself, is the first man to have every gone on intermittent hormone blockade. The benefits to being off hormone blockade are substantial. In Bud's experience sexual function returns 90 to 120 days after going off blockade, and other side effects from the medications resolve as well.

January 12, 2000, was the 10th anniversary of Bud's intermittent hormone therapy. On that day he was back on therapy, taking Lupron shots and Casodex (biclutamide) pills. Bud is not certain exactly how much time he has been off hormone blockade during the entire 10 years; he'd have to go back through all his records to be sure. But he does know that it's been a significant amount of time.

Intermittent hormone blockade has many potential advantages over continuous hormone blockade. With continuous blockade, men are often impotent, and suffer decreased sexual libido, muscle wasting, hot flashes and other side effects. By taking hormone blockade intermittently men can recover from these side effects when they stop the medications.

In some studies, doctors have treated men with double hormone blockade until their PSA level dropped as low as it will go, then the men were taken off hormone blockade and their PSA level was monitored.

The goal is to allow the men to recover from hormone blockade while off the medications. Once the PSA level rises to some arbitrary level, hormone blockade is started again. There are some studies that suggest that intermittent therapy may work just as well, or even better, than continuous therapy. An additional benefit of intermittent hormone blockade is that it is cheaper than continuous blockade.

Unfortunately for the sex drive, all men don't recover normal testosterone production once hormone blockade is stopped (although this may be beneficial as far as the cancer is concerned). In one study only 73 percent of the men had return of normal testosterone levels in the off treatment cycles.

The bottom line is that for many men, hormone blockade, or intermittent hormone blockade, may offer the most flexible treatment option.

Urologists have not always been supportive. "What the hell are you trying to do?" one urologist asked Bud, "Bankrupt urologists?"

"What do you mean?" Bud asked.

"Do you know that every time a man goes on these medications there's a loss of $20,000 to $30,000 to the doctor and the hospital?" In other words, no surgery!

Bud, an extremely likable and decent man, who believes that patients come first, was pretty offended by the urologist. He replied, "Doctor, I'll never use your name, but

I'll sure use your story." However, Bud points out that this was only one physician, and many hundreds since then are using hormone blockade with good results.

Ten years after starting intermittent hormone blockade, Bud Irish is winning tennis tournaments in Florida, where he has a winter home. Bud speaks to men all over the country about hormone blockade, and to keep his message pure, he doesn't own a single share of stock in any company that makes hormone-blocking medication.

Bud's was a bad case to start with. Over time, his objective came to be to live without surgery or radiation, and to prove IHT could be used successfully to wipe out prostate cancer. Bud will tell people what he did, but doesn't want to tell others what to do.

Bud Irish and several other heroic men with prostate cancer are profiled in a book, which many men and women will want to read called, *Prostate Cancer: Portraits of Empowerment*, edited by Nadine Jelsing and Paul Georgeades.

Intermittent Hormone Blockade and PSA Levels

Stephen Strum and Mark Scholz, two oncologists who regularly discuss prostate cancer on the Internet, have reported that if the PSA level on combined hormone blockade drops to less than 0.05 and stays there for at least 12 months, men are able to go off hormone blockade for two years. Men whose PSA levels do not drop so remarkably can only go off blockade for shorter periods.

There is a big difference in how well men do on intermittent hormone blockade depending on whether men have localized or metastatic prostate cancer. Those with localized cancer do better. One prospective, randomized, study called the RELAPSE study has been started to compare intermittent androgen blockade versus continuous androgen blockade in men who have relapsed after radical prostatectomy. Someday, the RELAPSE study and other controlled studies will tell us if and when we should be using intermittent androgen blockade.

It is hoped that intermittent hormone therapy might prevent the emergence of hormone resistant prostate cancer, although this has not been proven. Quite the contrary is possible, that at each cycle when the prostate cancer returns, it will come back faster and more aggressively each time. Right now, investigators hope that the opposite is true. The one thing intermittent hormone blockade clearly does is decrease the side effects by giving men a rest from the medications. This alone makes this avenue of investigation worthwhile. Eventually, randomized controlled studies will tell us if intermittent hormone blockade is a valuable new treatment modality. It is hoped that intermittent blockade will prolong life and increase the quality of life for men.

PSA Drop

When hormone blockade is utilized, if the PSA test drops to less than 4ng/ml within 24 to 32 weeks of treatment, men have an average life expectancy of almost 3 and 1/2 years. When the PSA fails to drop below this level within 24 to 32 weeks, men usually have an average life expectancy of about 18 months. Fortunately, a majority of men respond as in the first scenario. Such men are also then candidates for discontinuing hormone blockade in some study protocols until a rise in the PSA mandates going back on it again. Patients who respond positively may go off the hormone blockade for several months to over a year before a PSA rise suggests the need to go back on again. Then the cycle can be repeated as long as response occurs.

What Happens if You Wait Until Metastases Appear to Undergo Hormone Blockade?

Waiting until symptoms appear is a valid course of action for prostate cancer, but men should follow this area of the medical literature very carefully, because studies are ongoing and concepts are changing rapidly.

It's a very serious situation. According to urologist Thomas Stamey, once prostate cancer metastasizes to the bones, even with hormone blockade, about 50 percent of men will live for three years, about 31 percent will live for five years, and only 10 percent will live for at least 10 years.[93]

Are Urologists Good at Hormone Blockade Therapy?

Since urologists focus on surgery there is suspicion that they don't know how to give hormone blockade therapy well. Hank Porterfield, former president of Us TOO International Inc., has written that:

> "Surprisingly, urologists reported that they would recommend complete hormonal therapy to less than half of their patients with advanced disease (Stage D) with life expectancies of ten years or more. Only four in ten (40%) would be very likely to recommend complete hormonal therapy for permanent use immediately upon diagnoses of Stage D, and even fewer (36%) would be very likely to recommend it for all of their Stage D patients."[94]

---

[93] Stamey, TA: Prostate Cancer: Who Should be Treated? *Oncolink.* 1995. Available at:
http://www.oncolink.upenn.edu/disease/prostate/treatment/stamey.html.

[94] Henry A. Porterfield: Introduction from the Chairman of Us TOO International Inc. Prostate Cancer Support Groups. Louis Harris Survey, Perspectives on Prostate Cancer Treatments: Awareness, Attitudes and Relationships—A Study of Patients and Urologists. Available at http://www.ustoo.com/louis.html 1995. Quoted with signed, written permission of Us TOO and Louis Harris & Associates.

My own perspective is that urologists consider themselves surgeons and want to deal with patients who need surgery. Once a man is not a surgical candidate I would rather see him in the hands of an oncologist or other specialist who won't be disappointed if an operation isn't looming on the horizon. Hormone blockade entails a commitment to years of medical therapy and follow-up.

The Side Effects of Combined Hormone Blockade

The "flare reaction" from giving the testicle-blockers (LHRH agonists) has already been described. There are numerous other side effects from hormone blockade. For example, A large proportion of men experience hot flashes after surgical castration or treatment with LHRH agonists (medical castration).[95]

The blocking of male hormones can make men lose weight because their muscles will atrophy. Men will become impotent and their genitals will shrink. Some men will complain of the testicles becoming softer and smaller. There is concern that these changes in sexual libido and erectile function will become permanent if a man is on these medications too long.

One expert gives a warning that if you give hormone blockade for nine months or more, sexual function probably won't return to normal, while if you give it for four months or less, sexual function probably will return.[96]

Men can also suffer diarrhea, insomnia, liver damage, and, possibly, harmful effects to their cardiovascular systems. Numerous other side effects can occur, including nervous and twitchy legs, headache, and profuse sweating. Hormone blockade is not a pleasant experience. Stephen Strum, an oncologist specializing in prostate cancer, describes it like this:

---

[95] National Cancer Institute NCI/PDQ Physician Statement: Prostate cancer - Updated 03/97.

[96] Smith, Philip H: Carcinoma of the prostate: Case against immediate hormonal therapy, Mediconsult.com Limited. Available at http://www.mediconsult.com.

"ADT (androgen deprivation therapy) or hormone blockade is very difficult for many men. It is not a panacea as some would make it out to be. But, it is a damn effective modality for killing prostate cells. Unfortunately, ADT is associated with a spectrum of signs and symptoms (the androgen deprivation syndrome or ADS). Men undergoing ADT often experience problems with muscle atrophy, bone loss, decrease in size of the testicles and penis, decline in neuronal function with cognitive impairment, hair loss in some parts of the body, mood swings, vascular instability (hot flashes), anemia, and other problems. Physicians and patients must appreciate not only the anti-cancer effect of ADT but must also be aware of how androgen deprivation interacts with virtually every tissue in the male body.

"Therefore, it is essential that physicians employing ADT use approaches to prevent or remedy such untoward side effects. In fact, this is the foundation of all good medicine where the therapeutic ratio (benefit to the patient) is enhanced by improving the efficacy of treatment while decreasing adverse effects.

"Thus, in the setting of ADS, work-arounds (solutions) such as exercise, bisphosphonates, bone supplements, erythropoeitin, cognition enhancers and other means to support the patient are critical to a strategy of success."[97]

---

[97] Strum, Stephen B. E-mail to the author. August 19, 2004. Used with permission.

Hormones are tremendously important to our health. Oncologist Stephen Strum and other have coined the term "androgen deprivation syndrome" as a name for the consequences of hormone blockade, which include anemia, mental dysfunction, weakness, sexual dysfunction, and so on. The anemia often needs to be treated with erythropoietin (a drug that increases red blood cells). Men who are not aware that anemia can be a side effect may find their doctors doing painful bone marrow examinations and colonoscopies when all along their anemia is from hormone blockade therapy.

Dr. Robert Leibowitz and Triple Hormone Blockade®

Oncologist Robert Leibowitz deserves special mention. He believes that all local therapies such as the radical prostatectomy, cryoablation, and radiation are doomed to failure because prostate cancer is a systemic disease, not a localized one. In other words, if you have the kind of prostate cancer that is going to kill you, it has already escaped the prostate by the time you are diagnosed and obtain local therapy. Dr. Leibowitz invented triple hormone blockade® followed by finasteride maintenance®, and he owns the trademarks for both terms.

Triple hormone blockade® consists of a testicle-blocker, adrenal-blocker, and prostate-blocker. Dr. Leibowitz recommends Lupron, three pills of Casodex per day at one time, and one Proscar (finasteride) daily for 13 months and then keeps men on Proscar alone for maintenance.

Dr. Leibowitz has reported that he has treated over 150 men with clinically localized prostate cancer with triple hormone blockade® followed by Proscar maintenance. He also reports using his therapy on hundreds of men with more advanced prostate cancer. Dr. Leibowitz's rationale for treating men with triple hormone blockade® makes sense in terms of chemistry. In my last interview with him, Dr.

Leibowitz reported having over 99 percent prostate cancer-specific survival with triple hormone blockade®.[98]

I have interviewed several men diagnosed with localized prostate cancer who chose to undergo triple hormone blockade®. These men generally saw the radical prostatectomy as barbaric surgery, and viewed external beam radiation as too drastic as well. Many of these men had observed what a radical prostatectomy or radiation had done to someone else. The men I interviewed understood that the survival statistics attending surgery and radiation are not dramatically convincing, yet found it too passive to undergo watchful waiting until symptoms developed. These men started triple hormone blockade® up front. Most of these men are following their PSA level every month or every two months.

As with single and double hormone blockade, men on triple hormone blockade® are turned into "eunuchs" for the period that their testosterone is blocked. They lose their sexual desire and ability to have erections. For some men it is possible that the decline in sexual function will be permanent while for most others it will recover. Dr. Leibowitz reports that most men have recovery of normal testosterone levels within three to six months after stopping the testicle-blocker and the adrenal-blocker even while remaining on Proscar maintenance.[99]

Triple hormone blockade® up front is an option worth thinking about. As one of these men told me, you can always go back and get surgery, but you can't undo a radical prostatectomy. Dr. Leibowitz has reported his data about 150 men in a peer-reviewed medical journal.[100]

Men need to follow the literature on ideas such as triple hormone blockade® followed by Proscar maintenance.

---

[98] Leibowitz Robert, telephone interview with the author, November 15, 2004.
[99] Leibowitz Robert: I am the only one you are afraid to believe. *Cancer Communication.* 2000;16(3):6-9.
[100] Leibowitz RL, Tucker SJ: Treatment of localized prostate cancer with intermittent triple androgen blockade: preliminary results in 110 consecutive patients. *Oncologist.* 2001;6(2):177-82.

Doctors are producing new studies almost weekly on the permutations of hormone blockade.

The State of the Research

Fernand Labrie first described the use of combination hormone blockade in 1983. Over 20 randomized controlled studies on hormone blockade have been completed since then. Why haven't treatment outcomes been better sorted out by now? The reason is that there are so many questions, such as timing, duration, dose, and combination of hormone blockers, stages of cancer, continuous or intermittent therapy, or combination therapy with radiation or surgery.

Here is a quote from Dr. Labrie:

> "To date only continuous hormone blockade has been shown to prolong life in both local and metastatic prostate cancer. In localized disease, treatment with CHB for three years has been shown to prolong life, and with metastatic disease some men are kept on it for the rest of their lives as long as it continues to hold the cancer at bay."

For myself, your author, when the time comes, I am most interested in triple hormone blockade followed by Proscar maintenance, or in intermittent hormone blockade, as those therapies promise the highest quality of life. I will be following new studies on hormone blockade very carefully. I will close with a quote from Dr. Labrie who says:

> "With the proper use of the available diagnostic techniques and treatments applied without delay at time of diagnosis, death from prostate cancer should be rare. As a general but essential observation, it should be remembered that androgen blockade is the only

treatment shown in randomized clinical trials to prolong life in prostate cancer and, most importantly, this success has now been achieved at both the localized and advanced stages of the disease. Such data provide good reasons to suggest that androgen blockade, in addition to remaining the first-line treatment of advanced disease, should now be considered as an even much more efficient treatment of localized disease; endocrine therapy should thus be part of the therapeutic plan of any patient treated for prostate cancer at any stage of the disease. Localized prostate cancer is exquisitely sensitive to combined androgen blockade and patients should be able to take optimal advantage of this therapy alone or in combination with surgery or radiotherapy. Future research should permit us to eliminate the side effects of hormone therapy and further improve its efficacy but the presently available endocrine therapy is extremely efficient and well tolerated. Endocrine therapy certainly permits men to live longer and for many of them who are treated early, cure is a possibility."[101]

---

[101] Labrie, Fernand: Letter to the author. October 4, 1999. Quoted with signed, written permission.

Radiation Therapy for Prostate Cancer

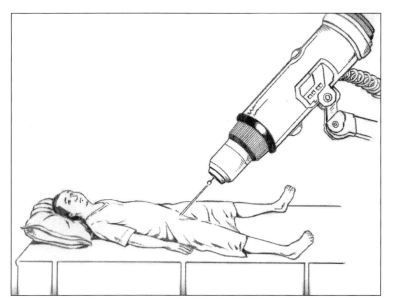

Figure 15. With external beam radiation the prostate is bombarded with photons. (Artist: Ramie Balbuena)

Introduction

External beam radiation therapy (XBRT) for prostate cancer began at Stanford University in 1956. It's called external beam radiation because the radiation is beamed from a machine that is outside, external to your body, into your body.

By the 1970s XBRT was the primary therapy for prostate cancer, but the invention of the modern version of the radical prostatectomy in the early 1980s, combined with a lot of false claims, caused the pendulum to shift towards surgery. Today the pendulum is shifting back toward radiation therapy, because there are now many different forms of radiation therapy, and there have been so many technical improvements in delivering radiation. This chapter is going to focus on traditional or "classic" external beam radiation therapy (XBRT).

A linear accelerator produces the radiation for XBRT. It's called a linear accelerator because the machine accelerates sub-atomic particles and slams them into metal. The metal then releases photons that are shaped into a beam. Photons are packets of energy.

Photon radiation is all around you. How it behaves depends on how much energy is in the photons. X-rays, sunlight, microwaves, and radio waves are all forms of photon radiation. It's just that the photons in x-ray radiation have so much energy that they can penetrate through the human body while sunlight, for example, affects only the surface of our body.

To treat prostate cancer with XBRT, photon beams are sent through the body into the prostate. This radiation kills cancer cells by damaging their DNA. Because cancerous cells divide more rapidly than normal cells, their DNA is more often in the state of division, which is when cells are most susceptible to radiation. In addition, normal cells are better at repairing themselves after radiation than cancerous cells are. One of the great advantages of XBRT is that it preferentially attacks cancer while being less damaging to normal tissue. With XBRT treatment of prostate cancer, men typically will undergo 28 to 40 radiation treatments over a period of six to eight weeks. Men lay on a table and the radiation is beamed into their prostate from several different angles during each treatment.

It's unfortunate that XBRT radiation sometimes damages normal tissue as well as cancerous tissue as it travels along its path to the prostate. On the other hand, XBRT is not major surgery and has fewer side effects across the board compared to the radical prostatectomy. The one problem somewhat unique to radiation therapy is bowel injury. Since the prostate is separated from the rectum by only millimeters, and the radiation beam cannot be perfectly focused (in fact it tends to bounce and scatter inside the body) XBRT can damage or irritate the rectum. Fortunately this side effect is becoming rare as radiation techniques improve.

Radiation works better the smaller the size of the tumor, because the smaller the cancer, the more focused the radiation beam can be. The more focused it is, the less likely it is that normal tissue will be injured. Small cancers are more likely to be killed as higher doses of radiation can be given to a smaller tumor than to a larger one.

XBRT radiation can be focused on the margins around the prostate as well as on the pelvic lymph nodes that lead away from the prostate. Thus XBRT might destroy cancer that would be left behind by the radical prostatectomy.

If external beam radiation therapy should fail, it's considered problematic to then have a radical prostatectomy. Operating on tissues that have received radiation is difficult, because irradiated tissue does not heal well. In perverted salesmanship, I have heard of urologists turning this into a reason to have a radical prostatectomy instead of XBRT. Such doctors may tell you that if the radical prostatectomy fails you can always have radiation, but if you have radiation you can't then safely have a radical prostatectomy. Urologists shouldn't be focusing on ways to promote their type of treatment, but should focus on giving men the best opportunity for up-front, curative, treatment with the fewest side effects. In reality, we don't have controlled studies that prove whether radiation or surgery is better, and if radiation is going to be used after surgery fails why not start with radiation in the first place?

After XBRT the prostate specific antigen (PSA) level should drop, but should not go to zero because some normal prostate tissue will survive the radiation treatments. Exactly how far the PSA should drop is debatable. Many studies have concluded that the PSA should go below 1.5 ng/ml, while others suggest that it should drop below 1.0 ng/ml and stay there. The wisest course may be to follow your PSA levels, and be wary of three rises in a row.

Radiation or Surgery

The big upside to external beam radiation compared to radical prostatectomy is that it's not a major operation and there are fewer side effects. Impotence and incontinence are less likely with external beam radiation therapy than with the radical prostatectomy.

The argument is which is better at curing prostate cancer, XBRT or radical prostatectomy? It hasn't been proven in controlled studies that the radical prostatectomy works, thus comparing XBRT to the radical prostatectomy is almost an exercise in futility, yet that's what almost everybody does.

Proponents of XBRT say that if you control for the fact that urologists take the healthiest patients with the smallest tumors and with the lowest Gleason scores, that XBRT is clearly better than radical prostatectomy. XBRT is better, advocates say, because efficacy is similar and there are fewer side effects than with radical prostatectomy. Advocates of radical prostatectomy will argue that their operation is best. The shame of both specialties, urology and radiology, is that neither has done the proper controlled trials to show whether either therapy actually cures prostate cancer, or whether one is truly superior to the other.

It's true that XBRT patients often have more serious cancers than do men undergoing radical prostatectomy. In a 1997 study, patients who had either radical prostatectomy or XBRT were stratified according to their pretreatment biopsy Gleason scores and PSA levels. The authors found that at 2 years there was no difference in the relapse rate after the treatments as measured by the PSA test. The authors concluded that because of the "vast difference in morbidity" between the two therapies that it is unfortunate that studies have not stratified patients by PSA and Gleason score and compared treatments head to head.[102] In a large Medicare study published in 1995, the authors found that when accounting for cost, efficacy, and side effects that external beam radiation therapy "dominated" the radical prostatectomy.[103] One radiation oncologist wrote:

> ". . . when similar patient populations . . . are compared, the 5-, 10-, and 15-year results are similar with radiation therapy or prostatectomy."[104]

To be perfectly clear on the issue of external beam radiation therapy versus the radical prostatectomy, I called Dr. Gerald E. Hanks, the radiation oncologist who is the Chairman of Fox Chase Cancer Center. He maintains what is probably the largest database on such patients in the world. Dr. Hank's take on the situation:

> "There is no evidence that the results of expertly performed surgery or external beam radiation treatment are different."[105]

---

[102] D'Amico AV, Whittington R, Kaplan I, Beard C, Jiroutek M, Malkowicz SB, Wein A, and Coleman CN: Equivalent Biochemical Failure-Free Survival After External Beam Radiation Therapy or Radical Prostatectomy in Patients with a Pretreatment Prostate Specific Antigen of > 4-20 ng/ml. *Int J Radiation Oncology Biol Phys.* 1997;37(5):1053-1058.

[103] Barry MJ, Fleming C, Coley CM, Wasson JH, Fahs MC, and Oesterling JE: Should Medicare Provide Reimbursement for Prostate-Specific Antigen Testing For Early Detection of Prostate Cancer? Part IV: Estimating the Risks and Benefits of an Early Detection Program. UROLOGY. 1995;46(4):445-461.

[104] Hanks GE: Long-term control of prostate cancer with radiation. *Urologic Clinics of North America.* November 1996;23(4):605-616. P. 605. Quoted with signed, written permission.

[105] Hanks, Gerald E. Personal communication with the author. April 29th, 1999. Quoted with signed, written permission.

External Beam Radiation Therapy Side Effects

One 1994 literature review of 2,611 men listed what the authors thought was a low rate of complications with XBRT. There was a 0.2 percent incidence of mortality, a 1.9 percent incidence of severe side effects, a 0.9 percent incidence of incontinence, and a 40 to 67 percent chance of impotence at five years.[106]

The savvy reader will notice right away that the risk of incontinence is drastically lower with external beam radiation therapy than with the radical prostatectomy. However, just how often incontinence occurs after XBRT therapy varies widely in the literature. One of the largest studies every done, a study of Medicare patients, found that only seven percent of men after radiation therapy were wearing pads or clamps to deal with incontinence, while thirty-two percent of post-radical prostatectomy patients were wearing pads, diapers, or clamps for incontinence.[107] The Medicare study was a good one because men were asked about their incontinence directly; the information was not obtained second hand from their physicians.

Both the XBRT and radical prostatectomy camps will argue, however, that the Medicare survey rates for incontinence published in 1996 are too high, that both procedures have been improved, and that today's incontinence rates are lower.

---

[106] Shipley WU, Zietman AL, Hanks GE, Coen JJ, Caplan RJ, Won M, Zagars GK, and Asbell SO: Treatment Related Sequelae Following External Beam Radiation for Prostate Cancer: A Review with an Update in Patients with Stages T1 and T2 Tumor. *Journal of Urology.* November 1994;152:1799-1805.

[107] Fowler, Floyd J. Jr., Michael J. Barry, Grace Lu-Yao, John H. Wasson, and Lin Bin; Outcomes of External-Bean Radiation Therapy for Prostate Cancer: A Study of Medicare Beneficiaries in Three Surveillance, Epidemiology, and End Results Areas. *Journal of Clinical Oncology.* 1996 August;14(8):2258-2265.

What is the Impotence Rate after External Beam Radiation Therapy?

Although impotence is not as likely with XBRT as with the radical prostatectomy, it's still a significant problem. Remember that the radiation beam cannot help but pass through nerves, arteries, and veins that are important to getting an erection. One group of authors performed a meta-analysis (a grouping of several studies already done) and found that the probability of impotence after XBRT was 42 percent while the probability after radical prostatectomy was 85 percent.[108] A 1997 article found the impotence rate after XBRT to be 31 percent.[109]

Some studies have shown, however, that after 10 years the post-XBRT impotence rate approaches or equals the impotence rate after radical prostatectomy. It's as if XBRT causes the important nerves, arteries, and veins to age faster. This means that the lesser incidence of impotence after XBRT compared to radical prostatectomy may not hold up over a 10-year period. Many men, however, if forced to make the choice of having to give up sex to cure prostate cancer, would rather let it fade out over ten years than cease abruptly with surgery. In addition, Viagra, Cialis, or Levitra (the erection enhancing drugs) may be much more likely to work for men post-irradiation than post radical prostatectomy, because less structural damage is done by radiation.

A word of caution about sexual function after XBRT: just as in the studies on impotence after radical prostatectomy, there is often no clear agreement on what defines impotence. Two studies may use completely different definitions. It would be best to define several important

---

[108] Wasson JH, Cushman CC, Bruskewitz RC, Littenberg B, Mulley AG Jr, Wennberg JE: A structured literature review of treatment for localized prostate cancer. Prostate Disease Patient Outcome Research Team. *Archives of Family Medicine.* 1993 May;2(5):487-493.

[109] Robinson, John W., PhD, C. Phsyc., Marie S. Dufour, BA, Tak S. Fung, PhD; Erectile Functioning of Men Treated for Prostate Carcinoma. *Cancer.* 1997; 79:538-44.

categories of sexual dysfunction. Not only will XBRT or radical prostatectomy often lead to impotence (can't get a hard enough erection for intercourse), but also to fewer erections, more down time between erections, less desire for sex, poor penile sensation, problems with orgasm, and other impairments of sexual function.

Importantly, men should know that transurethral resection of the prostate (TURP) and radiation therapy for prostate cancer seem to have cumulative effects on the rate of impotence. If a man has a TURP for benign prostatic hyperplasia and then is subjected to XBRT, there is a much higher likelihood of impotence; as many as 50 percent of patients who undergo both these treatments are impotent soon afterwards.

External Beam Radiation Side Effects in the Woolf Study

Steven H. Woolf, a family practitioner who would be expected to be more impartial than radiologists or urologists, provided a list of side effects after XBRT for the *New England Journal of Medicine* in 1995. He provided a range for each expected complication as best as he could determine them.

He noted acute gastrointestinal or genitourinary complications in 3 to 67 percent of the patients after XBRT. There were chronic complications requiring surgery or prolonged hospitalization in 1 to 2 percent of patients. Anal or rectal complications occurred in 2 to 23 percent, impotence occurred in 40 to 67 percent, urethral or bladder complications occurred in 3 to 17 percent, and incontinence occurred in 1 to 3 percent. Death occurred in 0.2 percent of patients.[110] Again, radiation therapists would argue that there have been great advances in the technology since the Woolf study.

---

[110] Woolf, Steven H, MD, MPH: Screening for Prostate Cancer with Prostate-Specific Antigen. An examination of the evidence. *New England Journal of Medicine*. 1995 Nov 23;333(21):1401-1405.

Radiation after the Radical Prostatectomy

It's common to find positive margins after the radical prostatectomy; in other words, when the final post-surgery pathology report comes back it shows that not all the cancer was removed. What should be done with these men? Should they get XBRT as soon as they are healed from the operation? Should their PSA be followed, and if and when it rises should they then get XBRT? No one knows the answer to these questions for sure, but many urologists send their patients with positive surgical margins on for radiation therapy, and there is growing support for doing so. I have to wonder if men who end up getting two therapies wouldn't have been better served by undergoing radiation therapy alone. It seems like a tragedy to receive both therapies when XBRT probably should have been done in the first place. This situation arises because we cannot tell before surgery, with great accuracy, whether prostate cancer has escaped the prostate. It also occurs because urologists are sometimes too eager to do surgery.

The Landmark Bolla Study

Men need to understand a simple concept, which is that when radiation therapy is given, the smaller the size of the prostate the better. With a small prostate the radiation beam can be more tightly focused on the prostate. Thus there is less scatter and less risk of side effects. By giving men hormone blockade until their prostates shrink, the risk of side effects from radiation therapy will be lower.

But there's another, exciting, reason why hormone blockade may be given prior to radiation therapy. A 1997 landmark paper, a randomized, controlled trial, by Michael Bolla et al, (called the EORTC Study) looked at two treatment groups. One group of men with locally advanced prostate cancer (T3) was randomized to receive only XBRT; the other group was randomized to receive one month of double hormone blockade (goserelin and cyproterone acetate) and XBRT, followed by single hormone blockade (goserelin) for three years. The second group, the one receiving hormone blockade with their radiation did much better; their five-year survival was increased by 45 percent.[111] The increased survival shown in this controlled study is a landmark in prostate cancer treatment.

The Lawton Study

Another prospective, randomized, controlled trial looked at men with positive lymph nodes. Ninty-eight men received XBRT plus single hormone blockade with a testicle-blocker, while 75 percent received radiation alone, unless a relapse occurred, and then they received hormone blockade. Interestingly, with about five years of follow-up, the estimated progression-free survival was 55 percent for those treated with XBRT and hormone blockade up front, and was only 11 percent for those initially treated with XBRT alone. The study estimated that hormone blockade increased survival by 5 to 8 percent at five years.[112]

The Pilepich Study

A similar study looked at 977 men with positive regional lymph nodes or with local extension of their prostate cancer, who were treated with radiation and single hormone blockade with goserelin (Zoladex), or with

---

[111] Bolla M, Gonzolez D, Warde P, Dubois JB, Mirimanoff RO, Storme G, Bernier J, Kuten A, Sternberg C, Gil T, Collette L, and Pierart M: Improved Survival in patients with locally advanced prostate cancer treated with radiotherapy and goserelin. *New England Journal of Medicine.* 1997;337(5):295-300.

[112] Lawton CA, Winter K, Byhardt R, Sause WT, Hanks GE, Russell AH, Rotman M, Porter A, McGowan DG, DelRowe JD, and Pilepich MV: Adrogen suppression plus radiation versus radiation alone for patients with D1 (pN+) adenocarcinoma of the prostate (results based on a national prospective randomized trial, RTOG 85-31). Radiation Therapy Oncology Group. *Int J Radiat Oncol Biol Phys.* 1997;38(5)931-939.

radiation alone, unless a relapse occurred, then hormone blockade was started. The study has shown an increase in overall survival in men with high-grade (Gleason 8, 9, 10) tumors.[113]

Pilepich 1995

Studies are beginning to show an increased survival with the combination of radiation therapy and double hormone blockade. Four hundred fifty-six men who were treated between 1987 and 1991 were randomized to receive either external radiation beam therapy alone, or XBRT and double hormone blockade with goserelin acetate (Zoladex) and flutamide (eulexin). The double hormone blockade was started two months before radiation therapy and continued during the entire course of radiation treatments. These were men with large, palpable, prostate cancers greater than 25 centimeters squared in size, not necessarily confined to the prostate, as some men had tumors extending beyond the capsule and some men had cancer in the lymph nodes close to their tumors. The amount of radiation given was 65 to 70 gray. The first results from this study of men with large, locally advanced, prostate cancer were published in 1995.[114] There was a significant decrease in local progression of the cancer in men treated with double hormone blockade and there was significant improvement in progression-free survival in men so treated. Of interest to many men will be that the majority of men in each arm of

---

[113] Pilepich MV, Caplan R, Byhardt RW, Lawton CA, Gallagher MJ, Mesic JB, Hanks GE, Coughlin CT, Porter A, Shipley WU, and Grignon: Phase III trial of androgen suppression using goserlin in unfavorable-prognosis carcinoma of the prostate treated with definitive radiotherapy: report of radiation therapy oncology group protocol 85-31. *Journal of Clinical Oncology.* 1997;15(3):1013-1021.

[114] Pilepich MV, Krall JM, al-Sarraf M, John MJ, Doggett RL, Sause WT, Lawton CA, Abrams RA, Rotman M, Rubin P, Shipley WU, Grignon D, Caplan R, Cox JD: Androgen Deprivation with Radiation Therapy Compared with Radiation Therapy Alone for Locally Advanced Prostatic Carcinoma: A Randomized Comparative Trial of the Radiation Therapy Oncology Group. UROLOGY. 1995;45(4):616-623.

the study eventually reported return of sexual function. I contacted the study's lead author, Miljenko Pilepich, M.D, a radiation oncologist.[115] Dr. Pilepich has been involved in many good studies regarding radiation therapy with or without hormone blockade. It's believed that the worse the prostate cancer is, the more you need higher doses of radiation, and the more likely you are to benefit from hormone blockade.

Hormone Blockade Plus Radiation

Although they are not reporting the perfect cure, papers in support of combining hormone blockade with radiation therapy are causing an important shift in prostate cancer treatment. But questions still need to be answered. Was it the combination that was effective, or was it possibly just the hormone blockade alone that was effective? And if hormone blockade is effective in combination with XBRT, what should be the timing and duration of treatment?

Urologists Versus Radiologists

If you read the literature carefully, looking for innuendo, you can see that radiologists do not always feel that they are treated fairly by urologists. By and large, radiologists are given the sicker patients to work with. Urologists then compare the radical prostatectomy done on healthier patients with patients who received radiation therapy and conclude that the radical prostatectomy is superior to radiation therapy. In reality radiation therapy has fewer side effects and may be more effective than the radical prostatectomy according the evidence we have today.

The most unfortunate thing of all is that since urologists, as the gatekeepers for prostate cancer patients, did not start out doing randomized controlled trials on the

---

[115] Pilepich, Miljenko: Personal telephone communication with the author, July 20, 1999.

radical prostatectomy from the very beginning, radiologists have almost been forced to skip those trials also, instead comparing radiation therapy to the outcomes from poor quality radical prostatectomy studies. As a result, the science behind prostate cancer treatments remains poor today. The few proper studies that have been done, by the way, have largely been done by non-urologists.

I asked the American College of Radiology for a statement about how they feel about radiation therapy for prostate cancer, and received this statement from J. Frank Wilson, MD, chairman of the College's Commission on Radiation Oncology:

> "Clinical studies have shown that a variety of radiation therapy procedures are just as effective as surgery in treating prostate cancer and have fewer side effects than radical prostatectomy. External beam radiation has, for years, been an effective tool in treating prostate cancer. More recently, radioactive seed implants and external beam 3D conformal treatment also have been proven to be exciting, highly effective new options available to patients with early-stage prostate cancer. 3D treatment allows radiation oncologists to shape the radiation beams around the cancerous area, delivering a more concentrated dose while sparing normal surrounding tissue. With seed therapy, the seeds are implanted directly into the tumor."[116]

---

[116] J. Frank Wilson, MD: American College of Radiology, Chairman of the American College of Radiology Commission on Radiation Oncology in a letter to the author, 12/29/1998. Quoted with signed, written permission.

The Doses of Radiation

XBRT will kill prostate cancer if a high enough dose is given. The problem has always been giving enough radiation to prostate cancer to kill it, without doing unacceptable harm to the surrounding normal tissue. Conventional XBRT has usually been given in doses from 64 to 68 Gray (Gy), and sometimes into the 70 Gray range. A Gray is a unit of measurement of radiation. But as higher doses were tried, too many side effects occurred.

Conclusion to XBRT

In some ways, classic external beam radiation (XBRT) is yesterday's news, because of newer kinds of external beam radiation.

In the next chapter I will discuss three-dimensional radiation therapy, in which higher doses of radiation can be given with fewer side effects. And let me preface the next chapter by saying that I would never undergo classic XBRT, because I believe that the newer types of 3-dimensional external beam radiation, or radiation seed implants, are better and safer.

Classic XBRT is not obsolete; however, as it's sometimes the only form of radiation treatment available to men.

3-D Radiation for Prostate Cancer

Radiation oncologist Dr. Howard Sandler says:

> "I feel strongly, based on the available scientific literature, that the long-term outcome with 3D conformal external beam radiotherapy is equivalent to radical prostatectomy for prostate cancer treatment."[117]

Marvin Blumberg

In 1992, at age 66, Marvin Blumberg discovered that his PSA level was 7.5 during a routine physical. He and his doctor ignored the elevation as possibly normal for a man his age—something that few doctors would do today. In the fall of 1994 another routine physical revealed a PSA of 8.0. His urologist performed a biopsy and told Marvin that he had "a few cancer cells" in his prostate. Marvin did nothing to treat his cancer because of the lack of significance his doctor placed upon it. Then, in August 1996, his PSA level was measured at 14.7. His cancer was staged at T2b (it was felt to involve more than 50 percent of one side of the prostate), and his Gleason score was 6 (later upgraded to 7 by another pathologist).

Marvin sought out a physician who was not a prisoner of the old standard—surgery. Marvin has an excellent education for researching his options, since he holds a degree in chemical engineering. He was president

---

[117] Sandler, Howard: Letter to the author, November 16th, 1999. With permission.

and C.E.O. of Carlgen Inc. for 14 years, and was a WW II combat veteran.

Marvin underwent 3 months of double hormone blockade (Lupron and Casodex), and then underwent 3D-conformal radiation, receiving 81 Gray of radiation under the direction of Dr. Michael Zelefsky at Memorial Sloan-Kettering Cancer Center in New York. Almost four years later, Marvin Blumberg's PSA is less than 1.0 and he has not suffered any serious side effects.

Mr. Blumberg was willing to go into great detail about his sex life, because he says, "Most men are stampeded into surgery and then kiss their normal sex life good-bye."

Marvin describes his sex life now:

"The radiation does dry up the ducts which carries the seminal fluid. This takes awhile to reach complete dryness. In my case about a year. You must also remember that I am now 73 years old, and some reduction in ejaculate was probably to be expected anyway. Anyway—it reached zero.

"I still get a normal erection whenever I want. I have sex about 4-5 times/week and can have normal sex and an orgasm albeit without an ejaculation. A normal erection will last about 15-20 minutes.

"I have experimented with 100mgs of Viagra. It takes some practice to know how to use this and how long to wait. It might not work every time due to some variables I have not identified yet. No fatty foods, it usually is effective anywhere from one to two hours after ingestion. Of course you STILL have to be in the mood and have a good woman as a partner. Once I got the Viagra procedure down, I could maintain a world class, door bustin' erection for up to one hour. Remember my age now. Not bad! So, if I want sex for a half-hour or so, I just let things work on a natural basis. If I want to get into an extended and heated session (over one hour), I pop a Viagra and can go on and on like the Energizer Bunny!"

Marvin's comments are particularly important because while researching this book I found that many men could not get erections after a radical prostatectomy even with Viagra, while after being treating with various forms of radiation therapy other men could get Viagra-enhanced erections.

3-Dimensional

Traditional radiation therapy with photons, called external beam radiation therapy (XBRT), uses a single, wide beam of radiation to irradiate prostate cancer. The beam is on a rotating gantry so the beam can be given in several different planes. XBRT usually delivers radiation in the range of 64 to 68 Gray, with higher doses often causing too many side effects to be acceptable. A newer development is three dimensional radiation therapy, where a computer is used in combination with CT scan pictures of the prostate, to mold the radiation beam. Three dimensional radiation therapies rely heavily on the images of the prostate taken with CT scans. Such therapy is called conformal, because the radiation conforms to the shape of the prostate. Today, there are several types of 3-D conformal radiation therapy:

- 3-D conformal radiation with photons
- Intensity modulated 3-D conformal radiation with photons
- 3-D conformal radiation with protons
- 3-D conformal radiation with neutrons

The forms of three-dimensional conformal radiation are important new developments in treating prostate cancer. Radiation oncologist Dr. Anthony Zietman, who works at Massachusetts General Hospital, says:

> "When it comes to prostate cancer, I advise men to get 3-D conformal radiation of some kind: regular 3-D conformal, intensity modulated 3-D conformal, or proton 3-D conformal. Which of these types is superior for prostate cancer remains unknown until further studies are done. Although radiation therapy is becoming more and more precise, it is never risk free, although the side effects are usually less than those of the radical prostatectomy."[118]

What's very important to know is that radiation kills prostate cancer and, in general, the higher the dose of radiation given, up to a certain point, the better. One study showed that for each 1 Gray increase of radiation administered there was an 8 percent increase freedom from prostate cancer at five years based on PSA levels.[119] But as the dose goes up so does the risk of side effects. This is why 3-D conformal radiation is such a breakthrough; 3-D conformal kills cancer better, while keeping the side effect rate acceptable.

There is little question in my mind, based upon the literature I've reviewed and the experts I've interviewed, that 3-D conformal radiation is superior to "classic XBRT" for treating prostate cancer. Men should always choose 3D-radiation over the old standard of XBRT. The questions that most men really need to ponder are how many Gray of

---

[118] Anthony Zietman, MD: Telephone interview with the author 2/9/1999. Quoted with signed, written permission.
[119] Hanks GE, Hanlon AL, Schultheiss TE, Pinover WH, Movsas B, Epstein BE, Hunt MA: Dose Escalation with 3D conformal treatment: five year outcomes, treatment optimization, and future directions. *Int J Radiat Oncol Biol Phys.* 1998;41(3)501-510.

radiation to submit themselves to, and whether to undergo hormone blockade simultaneously with 3D-radiation therapy.

3-D Conformal Radiation with Photons

The first 3-D radiation therapy to come about was 3-D conformal radiation therapy with *photons*. This technique uses computers to deliver photons from three dimensions. The idea is to deliver high doses of radiation to the entire prostate while avoiding as much normal tissue as possible.

Three-dimensional conformal radiation typically has been administered in doses of from 67 to 79 Gray, although recently I have seen the dose elevated up to 81 Gray. Yet, the side effect rate usually drops significantly compared to the old standby of external beam radiation therapy (XBRT) in which only about 65 Gray may be given. One study found that the side effect rate dropped 40 percent with 3-D conformational radiation.[120]

As expected, the complications can be the same as those with external beam radiation therapy. In the short term, rectal discomfort, rectal urgency, diarrhea, urinary frequency, nocturia, urgency, and dysuria can occur. The late complications are gastrointestinal and urinary problems. There is also a significant rate of impotence: 30 percent at two years in a Memorial Sloan-Kettering Study.[121]

A randomized, controlled study has shown the side effects of conformal radiation therapy to be less than those of conventional external beam radiation.[122] This 1999 study

---

[120] Hanks GE: Long-term control of prostate cancer with radiation. *Urologic Clinics of North America*. November 1996;23(4):605-616.

[121] Leibal SA, Zelefsky MJ, Kutcher GJ, Burman CM, Kelson S, and Fuks Z: Three-Dimensional Conformal Radiation Therapy in Localized Carcinoma of the Prostate: Interim Report of a Phase 1 Dose-Escalation Study. *Journal of Urology*. November 1994;152:1792-1798.

[122] Dearnaley DP, Khoo VS, Norman AR, Meyer L, Nahum A, Tait D, Yarnold J, Horwich A: Comparison of radiation side-effects of conformal and conventional

done in the United Kingdom, involved 114 men randomly assigned to conformal therapy, and 111 men assigned to conventional radiotherapy. Both groups of men were given 64 Gray of radiation, which controlled prostate cancer equally at five years; however, there was a significantly lower incidence of inflammation of the rectum (proctitis) and bleeding in the men who received conformal radiation. This is very important, as the most dreaded side effect of radiation therapy for prostate cancer is rectal injury.

There are several sites doing 3-D conformal radiation with photons. It's important for men to seek out medical venues that have considerable experience with this evolving new technology. Just as some surgeons are more artful than others are, some radiation oncologists are far more skilled than others. Some of the sites performing lots of 3-D conformal therapy are the Fox Chase Cancer Center in Philadelphia, Memorial Sloan-Kettering Cancer Center in New York, Massachusetts General Hospital in Boston, and the University of Michigan Medical Center in Ann Arbor.

Some of the numbers generated in case studies (admittedly not the ideal study) involving 3-D conformal radiation therapy are astonishingly good. Of 160 men with nonpalpable (T1a, T1b, or T1c) prostate cancer treated with 3-D conformal radiation therapy at Fox Chase Cancer Center (with an average of 73 Gray) between 1990 and 1994, 86 percent had no evidence of disease at five years based on their PSA levels. Only 6 patients had what would be considered serious toxicity from the treatment.[123] Radiation oncologist Gerald Hanks says that: "It is clear that 3-D conformal treatment has a superior late morbidity profile."[124] In other words, 3D conformal radiation has fewer

---

radiotherapy in prostate cancer: a randomised trial. *The Lancet.* 1999;363:267-272.

[123] Horwitz EM, Hanlon AL, Pinover WH, Hanks GE: The treatment of nonpalpable PSA-detected adenocarcinoma of the prostate with 3-dimensional conformal radiation therapy. *Int J Radiat Oncol Biol Phys*: 1998;41(3):519-523.

[124] Hanks, Gerald E: Personal communication with the author. April 21, 1999. Quoted with signed, written permission.

long-term side effects than the older style external beam radiation. Dr. Hanks should know. He has treated 1637 patients with 3D CRT from the years 1990 to 1999.

The survival numbers with 3-D conformal can be very good, although they vary depending on the baseline PSA, stage, and Gleason score just as they do with any form of prostate cancer treatment.

Importantly, in men with a poor prognosis because their stage is high, their PSA is high, or their Gleason score is high, there is evidence that adding hormone blockade to 3-D conformal radiation is better for keeping them free of disease than 3-D conformal alone based on follow-up PSA levels.[125] Of course, any improved success achieved by initially combining the two therapies must be tempered by the increased side effect rate of adding together the two therapies.

Intensity Modulated 3-D Conformal Radiation

Intensity modulation is an enhancement to 3-D conformal radiation. Intensity modulated radiation therapy (IMRT) uses millions of tiny pencil-thin photon beams instead of one large beam passing through the body. In three dimensions, IMRT delivers the pencil-thin beams of radiation to the target. This allows even more radiation to be delivered to the target tissues with less damage to surrounding, normal tissue—a feat that should increase cancer-killing power. Several centers are now doing 3-D conformal radiation therapy with intensity modulation, including Memorial Sloan-Kettering in New York, and New England Medical Center at Tufts University.

---

[125] Anderson PR, Hanlou AL, Movsas B, Hanks GE: Prostate cancer patient subsets showing improved bNED control with adjuvant androgen deprivation. *Int J Radiat Oncol Biol Phys.* 1997;39(5)1025-1030.

3-D Proton Beam Radiation Therapy

A newer type of radiation therapy uses protons instead of photons. Proton beams are able to be better focused and deliver more of their energy at the end of the beam, thus doing less damage to normal tissue. Remember, XBRT and 3-D conformal radiation with photons shoot out massless photons (energy particles) at cancer. Protons, on the other hand, do have mass as well as electrical charge. Because of their mass and charge, protons can be targeted so that they stop inside the tumor. Thus, proton beams have less scatter than photon beams. Because of the theoretical ability to be more precise, proton beam therapy may offer an advantage over the radiation therapies discussed so far.

The Massachusetts General Hospital was the first to offer proton beam therapy. Their machine was adapted from one used for physics experiments in the 1970s. They are currently giving patients 75 to 79 Gray with proton beam therapy. MGH is building a new machine and facility to better serve patients.

Loma Linda University Medical Center in California, which is located 60 miles east of Los Angles, was the first center to design a proton machine specifically for patients. They treated their first prostate cancer patient in 1991. They use a synchrotron, a special particle accelerator, to produce the protons. Proton beam therapy is conformal 3-D therapy because they use computers and CT scans to deliver the protons from almost any angle. At Loma Linda, although they sometimes give patients proton beam therapy alone, they typically give prostate cancer patients *proton* treatments for three weeks, and then follow that up with five weeks of 3D conformal radiation with *photons*. A total of about 40 treatments are required and the typical patient goes five times per week for eight weeks. Out-of-town patients move to the area for their two months of treatment. There are furnished apartments available for rent and other accommodations.

Loma Linda, in a 1998 paper, reported their five-year follow-up of 643 men showing their overall clinical disease-free survival at five years to be 89 percent.[126] There was a correlation between PSA and survival, with patients with lower PSAs doing better, a finding that is often seen in prostate cancer studies. Although the theoretical advantages of protons over regular external beam radiation are significant, especially if the side-effect profile can be kept low, long-term studies are still not available. I wish I could cite several randomized, controlled studies on proton beam therapy, but it's still a relatively new technique.

Conformal Radiation Therapy with Neutrons

Neutron radiation therapy also needs to be mentioned. In theory, neutron radiation has its own special advantages. The mechanism with which neutrons kill cancer is much more direct than that of photons. Photons work better when they strike cancer cells that are dividing. Neutrons damage the DNA of prostate cancer cells, dividing or not, in a way that can't be repaired as easily as photon damage can. Neutrons have mass so they can be delivered directly into the tumor, stopping there, instead of passing through. Neutron radiation is "stronger" than photon radiation, depositing more energy, and thus fewer treatments are needed. Men often go only three times a week for four weeks. Neutron radiation has its own special unit of radiation called the neutron-Gray. There are only a few facilities offering neutron therapy in the United States. They include the University of Washington in Seattle; the University of California at Los Angeles; the Tumor Institute at the University of Texas; the Fermilab Neutron Therapy Facility in Batavia, Illinois; and Harper Hospital in Detroit.

---

[126] Slater JD, Yonemoto LT, Rossi Jr. CJ, Reyes-Molyneux NJ, Bush DA, Antoine JE, Loredo LN, Schulte RW, Teichman SL, and Slater JM: Conformal proton therapy for prostate carcinoma. *International Journal of Radiation Oncology Biology Physics.* 1998;42(2)299-304.

Neutron facilities are also available in Europe and South Africa.

The most important thing to know about neutron radiation therapy is that one controlled study has shown an increase in survival. Ninety-one men with locally advanced prostate cancer were randomized to receive either a combination of neutron and photon (mixed-beam) radiation or the standard XBRT with photons alone. The overall survival rate for the combination therapy that included neutrons at 10 years was 46 percent, while it was only 29 percent for photons alone.[127]

Another study has shown improved loco-regional control with neutron irradiation compared to conventional photon irradiation in treating locally advanced prostate cancer. The strange thing is that a randomized controlled study comparing straight neutrons to photons did not show an increase in survival, but did show that neutron therapy can cause increased side effects. In fact, at least one center has dropped neutron therapy because of its more drastic side effects.

Problems with neutron therapy are that the dose to be given needs to be worked out, the greater toxicity needs to be better quantified, and randomized controlled studies need to be done so that we can be sure the increased survival seen by combining the two therapies is indeed real.

It's currently thought that the combination therapy of photons and neutrons supplies the best benefit with the fewest side effects. It also appears that the skill with which the facility can administer neutron radiation may be very important.

Based on what I know today, I would only have neutron therapy if it were at a place with which it is administered in true 3-D fashion. I would only have the

---

[127] Laramore GE, Krall JM, Thomas FJ, Russell KJ, Maor MH, Hendrickson FR, Martz KL, Griffin TW, and Davis LW: Eight Years Experience with Neutron Radiotherapy in the Treatment of Stages C and D Prostate Cancer: Updated Results of the RTOG 7704 Randomized Clinical Trial. *The Prostate.* 1987;11:183-193.

combination therapy of neutrons and photons, and I would seriously consider this treatment only for large, locally advanced prostate tumors exactly like those studied in the randomized, controlled study.

The role for neutron therapy in smaller, lower-stage prostate cancers has not been well studied, and for now, I would lean toward other, better-studied radiation therapies for early prostate cancer. Questions remain such as whether hormone blockade should be added to the mix. More randomized controlled trials need to be done with neutron therapy if it continues to show promise.

Dr. David Beyer

I asked Dr. David Beyer, of Arizona Oncology Services, to put the different kinds of external beam radiation into perspective. He told me that most men need to change their outlook on radiation therapy. Many men remember the "old days" 15 or 20 years ago when a grandfather or father had radiation therapy, but the technology has grown by leaps and bounds since then. The side effects that used to occur are rarely seen today. People actually used to get burned by radiation therapy in years past, something that is unheard of today.

In the "old days," the standard external beam radiation for the prostate typically involved 2-4 shaped beams that converged on the prostate. The earliest machines had only one position and the patient would be radiated with a beam going straight down and then would flip over to get the second beam. For the past 3 decades, machines rotate around the patient and allow 4 beams to be shot at the patient. Dr. Beyer explained that while treating the prostate in this "crossfire" a large amount of normal tissue surrounding the tumor was routinely irradiated.

Then along came 3-dimensional radiation with the better shaping of the treatment fields and improved computer modeling. Six to 12 beams were used to target the prostate from multiple angles, instead of 4. With these 3-D conformal machines far more accuracy is available. With 3-D conformal radiation, when the prostate is treated only a small zone or "margin" around it receives a high dose of radiation.

Then along came intensity modulated radiation therapy (IMRT) in which men receive 50 to over a 100 tiny beams of radiation; "beamlets," they sometimes call them. With IMRT you can move the patient or the beam around. You can also change the intensity of the radiation beam. This allows "modulation" of the radiation. In addition, doctors can actually change the shape of the beam as the machine arcs around the patient with special collimators that open and close to match the shape of the area being irradiated. The collimators are under continuous computer control.

Dr. Beyer said, "With IMRT you can actually treat a doughnut on a plate without irradiating either the plate or even the doughnut's hole!" This degree of precision, unheard of just a few years ago, has the power to revolutionize the entire realm of cancer therapy.

Dr. David Beyer says if the PSA is less than 10 and the Gleason score is less than seven he will avoid hormone blockade unless the prostate is too large to be safely irradiated. When the PSA is greater than 10 he starts thinking about adding hormone blockade. When the PSA is greater than 20, the Gleason score is eight or above, or a large bulky tumor is present he definitely prefers to give hormone blockade with radiation.

These are all conclusions that are born out by today's medical literature.

A New Development

Dr. James Wong, at Morristown Memorial Hospital in New Jersey, has developed another radiation system that might be the most accurate yet. For treating prostate cancer, he uses a Siemen's made Primatom linear accelerator, and delivers intensity modulated radiation therapy (IMRT). What makes his system unique is that a diagnostic CT-scan can be done before every treatment, right on the same bed where the patient lies during the radiation delivery. In theory, combing the two, imaging and treatment, so closely together, provides better accuracy.

Conclusion

The exciting thing about the different forms of radiation therapy is that they already appear to work as well as radical surgery, and yet clearly have fewer side effects. Even more hopeful are the tremendous advances that keep being made with radiation therapy. The technology seems to have unlimited potential. Radiation therapy may someday approach the ideal we hope for where prostate cancer can be completely destroyed without significantly harming any normal tissue.

Today, every man with prostate cancer must seriously look at 3D-radiation therapy in all its forms and in combination with hormone blockade therapy.

Radiation Seed Implants (Brachytherapy)

Moe and Larry (from a few chapters ago) have gone through watchful waiting and active non-invasive therapy. They cannot get PC SPES because of the recall, and no one does cryoablation in their area because it is so poorly reimbursed. Moe and Larry start to study radiation seed implants.

History

In 1985, radiation oncologist John Blasko and urologist Haakon Ragde performed the first modern version of *permanent* radiation seed implants in the United States. Via needles inserted through the skin, they placed radioactive iodine seeds directly into the prostate under transrectal ultrasound guidance—a procedure also called brachytherapy.

Brachytherapy means "slow therapy." The seeds slowly release radiation over time. For example, when radioactive iodine-125 seeds are used, they keep emitting appreciable radiation for about twenty months.

Drs. Blasko and Ragde started a revolution in prostate cancer treatment. In fact, Dr. Ragde told me he quit doing radical prostatectomies in 1998. The national trend is that the number of radical prostatectomies performed is going down significantly each year, while the number of men undergoing radiation seed implants has nearly doubled each year for 3 years in a row. In fact, it looks like seeds will overtake every other therapy by 2002 or 2003 as the most popular prostate cancer treatment.

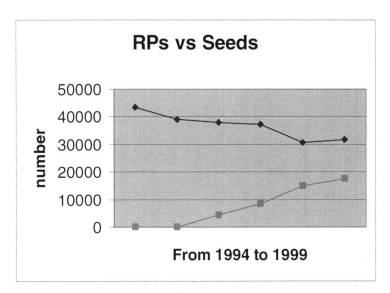

Figure 16. The graph shows that from 1994 to 1999 (Medicare Data) the number of radical prostatectomies per year (top line) has been going down, while the number of radiation seed implant procedures has been dramatically increasing every year (bottom line).

Blasko and Ragde now work at different institutions; Dr. Blasko is at the Seattle Prostate Institute and Dr. Ragde is at the Northwest Prostate Institute, also in Seattle, they have published many of the best studies on radiation seed implants. A radiation oncologist and urologist typically do the procedure jointly. Both types of specialists play important roles in doing seed implants and team care is very important. The radiation oncologist must plan the treatment and handle the radioactive isotopes, while the urologist typically places the needles into the man and provides the aftercare.

To find out more about radiation seed implants, I traveled to Dr. John Blasko's waiting room in Seattle, Washington. Two attractive women were sitting a few seats away. They were talking about their husbands who had prostate cancer. The first woman's husband was in the back seeing Dr. Blasko. Her husband had researched thoroughly, studying the material available on the Internet, and they had traveled from another state to see Dr. Blasko.

The husband, a dynamic-looking man of perhaps sixty years of age, soon appeared. As everyone in the waiting room talked, it quickly became apparent that the men coming to see Blasko were well-read. There was one major reason they were coming to find out about seeds: They didn't want to become impotent. These men had ruled out the radical prostatectomy because of its 100 percent rate of sexual dysfunction. These men, seeking seeds, intended to fight their cancer while maintaining their sexual function.

One Man's Story

After going to his fourth urologist, policeman John Smith,[128] was finally told that seed implants could treat his prostate cancer just as well as surgery. He canceled his radical prostatectomy.

He underwent palladium-103 seed implantation. After one day's sick leave he went back to work, where he endured some friendly ribbing about being radioactive.

Only a couple of months after the procedure, carrying his gun and pepper spray, he ran after a dangerous man who was possibly armed with an automatic weapon. The perpetrator had threatened to kill his wife and was a felon whose parole had been revoked; there was a warrant for his arrest. The felon was about 20 years younger than John.

John called in his chase, huffing & puffing, "Code 33, foot chase, southbound on 4th street, male, shaved head, gray sweat suit, 30 years old, muscular build, armed with a 22 automatic...."

John was thinking that if he'd had an RP (radical prostatectomy), he'd probably be incontinent under this much stress. He was thinking not only am I am not incontinent; I have no scar that hurts.

---

[128] John Smith is a pseudonym.

He captured the felon at gunpoint, sending him straight to prison for his parole violation.

Later, at his six-month follow-up after seeds he got his first PSA reading, which was down to 0.5. John was jubilant. His cancer appeared to be in remission and his lifestyle had not been destroyed by his prostate cancer treatment.

Why Seeds?

With external beam radiation therapy (XBRT), radiation has to pass through normal tissue to get to the prostate. It is this passage of the radiation beam through normal tissue that is responsible for most of the side effects of XBRT. To get around this problem, doctors came up with the idea of inserting radioactive seeds directly into the prostate. By implanting such seeds inside the prostate, higher doses of radiation can be delivered to the cancer, while keeping the dose of radiation to surrounding tissues to a minimum. The idea is to place the radiation only where it is needed—into the prostate itself. Indeed, the killing advantage of seeds is that their radiation is so focused within the prostate. Physicians can give higher, more lethal-to-cancer doses of radiation with less damage to surrounding healthy tissues.

Seed implantation has drastically improved with advances in computers, transrectal ultrasound, and CT scanning of the prostate. Not too long ago, the prostate was very carefully mapped out and then the seeds were placed. Today, the prostate can be mapped with computers during the procedure in real time while the seeds are being placed. The procedure keeps getting more accurate. In addition, sometimes ribbons of seeds embedded in plastic are now used instead of placing them one at a time.

Seed implantation is not major surgery. It can be done as an outpatient procedure, often under general anesthesia. Some men choose spinal anesthesia, so they are actually awake during the procedure, although they feel nothing in their pelvic area. Depending on the size of the prostate, 50 to 85 seeds may be put in. Each seed is so small that 10 or 12 of them laid in a circle would be about the size of a dime.

Radiation seed implants are put into the prostate through needles inserted into the perineum (the skin area between the testicles and anal opening).

Advantages

A significant reason why men choose radiation seed implants is reduced risk of sexual dysfunction compared to radical prostatectomy or external beam radiation. Both XBRT and RP damage nerves, arteries, and veins important for sexual function, while seeds tend to minimize this damage.

Three types of Radioactive Implants

There are three types of seed implants, iodine, palladium, and iridium. Iodine and palladium seeds are left inside the prostate, while iridium is removed from the body when treatment is finished. Each of these different isotopes has its advantages and disadvantages.

Iodine

Moe and Larry discuss it, and Moe chooses to go with Iodine seed implants. Iodine-125 (125 is the atomic weight) was the first isotope used and is still the most commonly used seed implant today. There is far more experience with iodine than with any other radioactive element.

Iodine-125 is perfect for Moe, because it's generally used for small cancers in small-sized prostates with low PSA levels.

Its half-life of radioactivity is about 60 days, and it takes about 10 half lives for its activity to disappear. It will slowly deliver radiation to Moe's prostate for about 20 months.

Palladium

Larry decides to go with Palladium. "I have a faster growing cancer than you, Moe," he says, "so I'll have the faster radiation seeds."

Larry knows that palladium-103 seeds emit radiation for about 24 weeks, instead of the 20 months for iodine.

Palladium-103, because it delivers higher energy during a shorter period of time, is often used for larger cancers with higher PSA levels, like Larry's. Although, there is little scientific proof against using it for any type of prostate cancer that iodine is used for.

Snuffy Meyers, MD

What does a cancer doctor do when diagnosed with prostate cancer? At age 55, Dr. Charles "Snuffy" Myers, a medical oncologist and Director of the Cancer Center at the University of Virginia was diagnosed with prostate cancer.

Dr. Myers was formerly a cancer doctor at the National Cancer Institute, which put him on a first name basis with many of the world's foremost cancer experts.

Snuffy's wife Rose got on his case, and Snuffy finally went in for an exam and a PSA test. His urologist found a rock-hard nodule on his prostate. His PSA was 20.4, and his biopsy revealed a Gleason score of 3+4=7.

Snuffy started on triple hormone blockade with Lupron, Casodex, and Proscar (finasteride) for three months. Then he underwent external beam radiation therapy and radioactive Palladium seed implantation by Dr. Michael Dattoli in Tampa, Florida.

In Snuffy's case the cancer had spread to one seminal vesicle and to his iliac lymph nodes, so the external beam radiation therapy was extended to cover those areas.

Dr. Meyers stayed on hormone blockade for 18 months. He also took Fosamax and Rocaltrol, two drugs which help prevent osteoporosis.

Dr. Meyers says this about choosing palladium over iodine:

> "Palladium has a shorter half life and a more focused (narrower) spread of radiation. Also the design of the palladium seeds make seed migration less likely. In other words, except for being cheaper, iodine has no advantages."[129]

Dr. Snuffy Myers is now an outspoken educator about prostate cancer and publishes an excellent newsletter. You can find out more, and can obtain his newsletter, at his web site www.prostatefocus.com. Dr. Meyers also runs a clinic devoted to prostate cancer, which he calls the American Institute For Diseases of the Prostate.

Iridium-192

Dr. Nasir Syed performed the first transperineal iridium-192 seed transplantation for prostate cancer in the United States. He did the procedure in 1977—eight years before Drs. Blasko and Ragde performed permanent seed implants.

The major advantage is that because iridium-192 delivers a rapid, high dose of radiation, the seeds can be removed at the end of the treatment session. No permanent seeds are left inside the body. This also means that the seeds can't accidentally move around inside your body as iodine or palladium seeds can do, perhaps accidentally irradiating the urethra or rectum.

---

[129] Meyers, Charles: Email to the author. April 18th, 2003. Quoted with e-mail permission.

For iridium-192 radiation treatments, catheters are usually placed inside the prostate and a machine puts the seeds in and then removes them several times—often three or four times—over a two-day period in which the man stays in the hospital. Then everything—seeds and catheters—are removed. The two days that a man must stay in the hospital have made iridium implants less popular with many physicians, because they have to provide two days of patient care compared to a couple of hours with iodine or palladium implants.

Iridium-192 radiation is released very quickly compared to the slow release of radiation by iodine or palladium. It is also fairly typical for iridium implants to be followed by external beam radiation therapy.

Choosing your Type of Seed Radiation

When should you use which seed? Conventional wisdom is that you can always use iodine, however, the perfect patient has a small cancer, with PSA less than 10, and Gleason score of six or below. There is some consensus about using palladium seeds for tumors with Gleason scores of 7 or higher. I found no clear rules about when to use iridium seeds, but men use them when they don't want any foreign bodies left inside of them. Nasir Syed, MD and Alvaro Martinez, MD, neither of whom I have met, probably have the most experience with iridium. There is a great deal of flexibility, including physician and patient preference involved in choosing a seed implant.

Hormones and Seeds

Sometimes radiation seed implantation is preceded by hormone blockade. Hormone blockade kills local cancer cells, possibly clears the body of any cancer cells outside of the prostate, and shrinks the prostate. It's easier to implant seeds in a small prostate than into a large one. Brachytherapists prefer the prostate to be less than 60 grams in size before doing the procedure. Larry has a big prostate, while Moe's is small. So Larry, undergoes hormone blockade prior to getting his seed implants, to shrink his prostate down to size, and hopefully, to kill any prostate cancer that might be outside his prostate.

External Beam Radiation Followed by Seeds

"I can't figure out if I should have seeds first, and then external beam radiation or the other way around," Larry moans to his friend Moe.

"We'll figure it out," Moe replies.

Why not lower the dose of the external beam used and then place radiation seed implants, creating a synergistic therapy? This is often done today. Many protocols start with external beam radiation and then seeds are implanted as a boost directly into the tumor. Because seeds are going to be done, a lower dose of radiation is given by external beam therapy, often only around 45 gray (instead of the typical 75 to 79 gray that might be given if a man was treated with 3-D external beam radiation alone).

Advocates state that not only is the combination good for local organ contained disease, but also that more advanced cancers can be treated this way, because by combining the two modalities radiation can be given to the prostate margins and pelvic lymph nodes, if required.

Seeds Followed by External Beam Radiation

The reverse can also be done: Radiation seed implants can be followed by external beam radiation. With this approach, the seeds are used as landmarks to focus the external beam radiation. This technique has been dubbed combined precision irradiation (CPI). Its leading proponent is Dr. Frank Critz of the Radiologic Clinics of Georgia. Dr. Critz believes that aiming for the seeds helps doctors deliver the external beam radiation more precisely and at lower doses.

The concept of CPI is made more attractive to many men, because the neurovascular bundle on one side (the side away from the cancer) is intentionally spared from radiation when it is thought to be possible to do so. This improves a man's chances of maintaining his sexual potency.

"I want one nerve bundle spared," Larry declares, when he finds out about this.

1998 Dr. Frank Critz

Dr. Frank Critz and his group at the Radiologic Clinics of Georgia, doing combined precision irradiation, showed that 72 percent of 1,020 men had a PSA level that did not rise after treatment with seeds followed by external beam radiation.[130] One study by urologist Patrick Walsh on the radical prostatectomy showed that 70 percent of men with clinically localized prostate cancer had an undetectable PSA level at 10 years after the surgery.[131] Thus, using these types of studies, where PSA is used as the end point instead of actual deaths from prostate cancer, and where statistical projections are made out to 10 years, these two treatments have essentially identical results.

The data bodes well for CPI. In fact, it may be the best of all worlds according to present data, resulting in the fewest side effects and the highest survival rate.

If combined precision irradiation is so great why aren't more men undergoing it? The reason is probably that few places are doing it, and it is difficult for the average patient to pack up and head for the Radiologic Clinics of Georgia to get seed implants, and then it's difficult to stay for all 30 external beam radiation treatments, which will be

---

[130] Critz FA, Levinson AK, Williams WH, Holladay CT, Griffin VD, and Holladay DA: Simultaneous radiotherapy for prostate cancer: 1251 prostate implant followed by external-beam radiation. *Cancer J Sci Am.* 1998;4(6):359-363.
[131] Walsh PC, Partin AW, Epstein JI: Cancer control and quality of life following anatomical radical retropubic prostatectomy: results at 10 years. *Journal of Urology.* 1994;152(5 part 2):1831-1836.

needed afterwards. Yet, in terms of survival and side effects, it might be well worth the trip.

Are seeds followed by radiation better than radiation followed by seeds? I don't know. I have not seen enough adequate studies to make a decision about which technique is best. The argument has been made that if the seeds are already in place, they may cause the external beam radiation to scatter and be less focused. At this time, I don't know which is best.

Follow-up

Some centers that perform radiation seed implants biopsy the prostate a year afterwards to make sure the cancer is gone, and all centers should follow the PSA level after treatment with seeds. It is hoped that following the PSA alone will prove to be sufficient so that repeat biopsies can be avoided.

Ideal Candidates

Anyone who is a candidate for surgery is also a candidate for radiation seed implants. Seeds in combination with external beam radiation and hormone blockade can also be used to treat men who have prostate cancer too advanced for surgery.

The ideal candidates for radiation seed implants as a single therapy are men with locally confined prostate cancer (stages T1 or T2). The smaller the cancer the better when it comes to using radioactive seeds alone. For seeds as a single therapy, doctors like to see low-grade (Gleason 2, 3, 4) or medium-grade (Gleason 5, 6, 7) cancers with initial PSA levels less than 10.[132] Indeed, commonly reported criteria for seeds alone include a Gleason score less than or

[132] Blasko JC, Ragde H, Luse RW, Sylvester JE, Cavanagh W, and Grimm PD: Should brachytherapy be considered a therapeutic option in localized prostate cancer? *Urologic Clinics of North America.* November 1996;23(4):633-650.

equal to seven, a PSA less than 10, stage T2a or lower, and a prostate less than 60 grams in size.

When the amount of cancer is larger, or the grade is higher, doctors look to add external beam radiation or hormone blockade, or both.

The current recommendations by the American Brachytherapy society are that men with a high probability of prostate-confined cancer be treated with radiation seed implants alone, while men with significant risk of extraprostatic extension of their cancer undergo seeds combined with external beam radiation therapy.[133] According to the Society, either Iodine-125 (dose 145 Gray) or Palladium-103 (Dose 115 Gray) can be used. If the prostate cancer is thought to be confined to the prostate, seeds alone are given. If it's not confined to the prostate, external beam radiation is given first, and a smaller dose of seeds is implanted.[134]

Picking a Brachytherapist

As with any prostate cancer treatment it is very important to pick an artist to do your radiation seed implants. Experience and outcomes vary widely. Poorly done seed implantation can be a disaster for men, while well-done seed implantation barely interrupts a man's life. When I wrote this, thirty-five doctors were doing nearly half of all the seed implant procedures being done in the United States. Some doctors perform 100 to 300 brachytherapy procedures per year. You should pick out a doctor who does lots of procedures and has an outstanding track record.

---

[133] Nag S, Beyer D, Friedland J, Grimm P, Nath R: American Brachytherapy Society (ABS) recommendations for transperineal permanent brachytherapy of prostate cancer. *International Journal of Radiation Oncology Biology and Physics.* 1999;44(4):789-799.
[134] Nag S, Beyer D, Friedland J, Grimm P, Nath R: American Brachytherapy Society (ABS) recommendations for transperineal permanent brachytherapy of prostate cancer. *International Journal of Radiation Oncology Biology and Physics.* 199;44(4)789-799.

Side Effects

Radiation seed implants can be pretty tame in terms of side effects as prostate cancer treatments go. The process is usually a single-session outpatient procedure. Side effects such as incontinence, impotence, and urinary stricture occur less often than with radical prostatectomy.

Palladium seeds usually cause urinary trouble within weeks, that, it is hoped, will resolve over a couple of month's time. Iodine seeds are lower energy and longer acting; they often induce urinary trouble a month or two after seeding, and the symptoms may last up to a year before resolving.

Physicians typically chose from a number of protocols to treat urinary trouble after seed implantation. Steroids, nonsteroidal anti-inflammatories, alpha-blockers, and urinary anesthetics such as phenazopyridine (Pyridium, Pyridiate, Urodine, Geridium) may be used.

Fewer side effects makes seeds popular among men being treated for prostate cancer. Men are slightly radioactive after radiation seed implantation until the radiation decays. They are usually told to avoid close contact with pregnant women or children for 2 months after seed implants, in fact, they are often told to stay at least six feet away. Men are usually advised to wear condoms during sex for three months because a radioactive seed could be ejaculated at orgasm, and it is sometimes recommended that men not sleep in the same bed with their sexual partner for two weeks or so depending on the type of isotope given. If a seed does come out during urination or sex, men are advised to flush it down the toilet, and not to directly touch the seed.

Expect pain, burning, stinging with urination, and frequency of urination at some point after the procedure. Urinary symptoms are one of the tradeoffs with seeds. Although more radiation can be given directly to the cancer than with 3D conformal radiation, which may mean better killing effect, there is also a greater likelihood of urinary symptoms. Urethral strictures occur in about 12 percent of cases. These problems vary with the type of isotope given. There may also be pain in the perineum, which may last for months. In some cases prostatitis symptoms may become permanent after seed therapy. Radiation seed implants are foreign bodies left behind in the body permanently, and they can sometimes continue to induce swelling and pain. The seeds can and do become dislodged over time. In one large study, 6 percent of men had a seed escape the prostate and travel to the lungs, although newer techniques with the pellets being implanted attached to Vicryl suture promises to reduce the rate of this side effect. In any event, seeds escaping to the lungs often do not cause symptoms.

One study showed the rates of complications in 71 men who had radiation seed implants to be mild proctitis (rectal swelling) in 4.2 percent and urinary retention in 5.6 percent, sexual potency deteriorated in only 6 percent, while no man suffered urinary incontinence.[135] Another study showed that at 5 years, 53 percent of men undergoing seeds suffered erectile dysfunction, while 43 percent of men undergoing 3D conformation radiation suffered erectile dysfunction.[136]

Side Effects of Combined Therapy

Combination therapy means more risk. Men need to be on guard, weighing those risks against the risk of not treating all their prostate cancer. A study from France[137] of

[135] Stone, Nelson N, MD, and Richard G. Stock MD: Brachytherapy for Prostate Cancer: Real Time Three-Dimensional Interactive Seed Implantation. *Techniques in Urology.* Vol 1, No 2, pp. 72-80. P 1. 1995.

[136] Zelefsky MJ, Wallner KE, Ling CC, Raben A, Hollister T, Wolfe T, Grann A, Gaudin P, Fuks Z, and Leibel SA. Comparison of the 5-Year Outcome and Morbidity of Three Dimensional Permanent Iodine-125 Implantation for Early-Stage Prostatic Cancer. *Journal of Clinical Onclology.* 1999;17(2):517-522.

[137] Joly F, Brune D, Couette JE, Lesaunier F, Héron JF, Pény J, and Henry-Amar M: Health-related quality of life and sequelae in patients treated with

71 men treated with temporary iridium implants that had external beam radiation, either before or after the radioactive implants, looked at the quality of life for men after the procedure. The amazing thing was how much more often patients would report side effects than their doctors would. Physicians reported urinary incontinence in 12 percent of cases while 40 percent of patients said they suffered from it. Physicians reported pelvic pain on only 5 percent of patients while 38 percent of patients reporting having such pain.

Some of the side effects noted by Dr. Critz and others are rectal inflammation, diarrhea, rectal bleeding, rectal ulcers, bladder inflammation, bloody urine, incontinence, urethral stricture, and urethral necrosis. These are all the same risks that are found with any form of radiation therapy to the prostate.

Outcomes

Dr. Michael J. Zelefsky, Chief of Brachytherapy and Associate Professor of Radiation Oncology, says:

> "The outcomes for 3-D conformal radiation therapy and brachytherapy for early stage prostate cancer are comparable to surgery. Because of improvements in technology, both radiation approaches can deliver high doses to the prostate, while minimizing the harm to surrounding normal tissues. The precision of both forms of radiation therapy results in less urinary incontinence than with surgery."[138]

---

brachytherapy and external beam irradiation for localized prostate cancer. *Annals of Oncology*. 1998;9:751-757.
[138] Zelefsky Michael J: Letter to the author December 16, 1999. Quoted with signed, written permission.

Advocates believe that radiation seed implants can send prostate cancer into remission with fewer side effects than the radical prostatectomy. The problem is that there are no controlled studies comparing survival after seeds to surgery or to watchful waiting. Instead the data we have is generally from case series studies. A case series study is simply an observational study of a group of men. A case series does not have a control group. These types of studies do not actually prove that one procedure is better than another; only controlled studies can do that. We are left with this situation of comparing case series studies for one treatment against the other, which is a very imprecise and unfortunate situation.

PSA after Seeds

Undergoing treatment with seeds will dramatically lower the PSA level. The PSA level is then followed over time, every 3 months or 6 months at first, then at least every year. As long as the PSA stays level everything is considered fine. If the PSA level rises three times in a row, then everyone becomes suspicious that the cancer may have returned. At about 18 months after treatment many men experience a bounce in their PSA, where it rises and then falls, but this may have no long term importance and is apparently just due to healing of the prostate.

Aubrey Pilgrim

Aubrey Pilgrim, a member of the Mensa high IQ society, was a doctor of chiropractic when he went back to school and studied electronics. He helped to assemble the world's first video recorder. After retiring from Lockhead, he went on to write books such as: *Build Your Own IBM Compatible and Save a Bundle.* Over 500,000 copies of his books have been sold.

Aubrey Pilgrim was sixty-seven when his prostate cancer was discovered. His PSA was 10.2 and his Gleason score was 3+2=5. Two urologists recommended a radical prostatectomy, which he underwent. The operation did not go well; he required six units of blood. Afterwards, Pilgrim became impotent and incontinent. He developed Peyronie's disease, a seldom mentioned but surprisingly frequent side effect of the radical prostatectomy that causes the penis to curve in a painful manner. Pilgrim reports that he has fantasized about shooting his urologist in the groin so that his urologist would suffer the same symptoms as he does.

Pilgrim reports that if he were diagnosed with prostate cancer today he would chose radiation seed implant therapy rather than mutilating surgery. He wrote the book: *A Revolutionary Approach to Prostate Cancer,* which explains many of his opinions about prostate cancer. Over 20 physicians contributed to his book.

Pilgrim describes attending various prostate cancer support groups in the Los Angeles area. Inevitably, someone would get up and ask how many men were sexually potent after the radical prostatectomy. Usually only three or four out of 50 or 60 men (about 6 percent) would raise their hands. Today, Pilgrim has a lot of trouble believing what his urologist told him before his surgery, that there was only a 50 percent chance he would become impotent from his radical prostatectomy.

MRI-Guided Prostate Brachytherapy

As this book was going to press, I learned of a new brachytherapy technique. One center is doing MRI (magnetic resonance imaging) guided brachytherapy instead of the usual TRUS (transrectal ultrasound) guided brachytherapy and has published spectacular results.

Harvard Radiation oncologist Anthony D'Amico has published that MRI-guided brachytherapy, as a minimally invasive procedure, works just as well as the radical prostatectomy without all the side effects of major surgery.

D'Amico's study involved 196 patients with localized prostate cancer, clinical Stage T1c, a PSA level less than 10 ng/mL, and Gleason scores of 7 (3 + 4) or less.[139]

Final word

Don't expect your urologist to know all about seeds. To really get the lowdown on seeds, in my opinion, you typically need to see a radiation oncologist.

Importantly, based on medical studies, I firmly believe that any prostate cancer that can be treated by surgery can be better treated by radiation seed implants. In addition, prostate cancers that are too advanced for surgery can still be treated with seeds in combination with hormone blockade and external radiation.

Moe had a small prostate cancer, stage T1(c), with a low Gleason score of 3 + 2 = 5, and a PSA of 8. He underwent seeds by an experienced brachytherapist and was very satisfied with his result.

Larry's numbers were more worrisome. He was stage T2(a) – a lump could be felt, his Gleason was 3 + 4 = 7, his cancer was bigger with two cores being positive, and his PSA was 16. He also had a large prostate. Larry underwent much more intense therapy, having hormone blockade, 3-D conformal external radiation, and seed implants. He was also willing to risk more side effects in order to be satisfied that he had done everything he could for his prostate cancer.

---

[139] D'amico AV, Tempany CM, Schultz D, Cormack RA, Hurwitz M, Beard C, Albert M, Kooy H, Jolesz F, Richie JP: Comparing PSA outcome after radical prostatectomy or magnetic resonance imaging-guided partial prostatic irradiation in select patients with clinically localized adenocarcinoma of the prostate. Urology. 2003 Dec;62(6):1063-7.

The Radical Prostatectomy

> "The hallmark of medical professionalism is putting the needs of patients above one's own."[140]

> ". . . the surgeon who operates needlessly, as it were, possesses the morality of a rapist."[141]

> ". . . many decisions are based on patients' hopes and physicians' professional preferences instead of on any solid knowledge of what will happen to the patient."[142]

Men's reactions to prostate cancer vary, but I couldn't help noticing that the response of actor John Wayne's character in the movie *The Shootist* is typical. John Wayne, a gunfighter in the year 1901, goes to see actor Jimmy Stewart, who plays the town doctor:

Jimmy Stewart: You don't trust my profession.

---

[140] Koop, C. Everett: Medicine Man: A pioneering pediatric surgeon recalls his early days in medicine, when doctors were gods among men. PEOPLE. March 29, 1999. Pages 77-80. p. 80. Quoted with signed, written permission from PEOPLE.

[141] Ron E. Losee, MD: *Doc: Then and Now with a Montana Physician*. New York: Ivy Books. 1994. Quoted with signed, written permission.

[142] David Eddy, MD, PhD: Telephone conversation with the author 12/08/1998. Quoted with signed, written permission.

> John Wayne: In my profession you don't trust too much or you won't see too many birthdays.
> Stewart: Bend over the table there . . . trap-door down. (Jimmy Stewart does a rectal exam on John Wayne off-screen and then they look at each other.)
> Wayne: Why don't you just say it flat out?
> Stewart: All right. You have a cancer. Advanced.
> Wayne: Can't you cut it out doc?
> Stuart: We'd have to gut you like a fish.[143]

John Wayne's character, who has prostate cancer, mirrors the reaction of most men when they first learn that they have it: "Cut it out, doctor!" The problem in 1901 was that because the prostate is so deep inside the pelvis, so locked up with other important structures, that to try to remove it, did indeed "gut men like a fish."

Eventually, instead of letting men die from advanced prostate cancer without doing anything, a non-lethal operation was invented, which was called the radical prostatectomy. Urologist Hugh Young first performed it in 1904, leaving all his patients impotent and incontinent. He emasculated them of the nerves, arteries, and veins, which they needed for sexual potency, and savaged them of their urinary sphincters. Dr. Young did "gut men like they were fish." Morbidity was high.

Seventy-eight years later, urologist Patrick Walsh invented today's version of the radical prostatectomy. He invented modifications resulting in a less bloody operation, which allows for the option of sparing two nerve trunks, but not their branches, which are important for normal sexual function. Dr. Walsh performed the first modern version of the radical prostatectomy on April 8th, 1982. Dr. Walsh

---

[143] The Shootist. Paramount Pictures. Los Angeles 1976. Directed by Don Siegel. Produced by M. J. Frankovich and William Self; Dino de Laurentis / Paramount.

personally performed 820 radial prostatectomies between 1982 and 1990, and continues to do them every year.

Despite improvements in its technique, even today, the radical prostatectomy is major surgery. It's also one of the most controversial operations in the history of medicine.

Dr. Walsh introduced the phrase "anatomical approach to the radical prostatectomy" to describe his version of the radical prostatectomy. He considers it "anatomical" because by better knowing the anatomy, surgeons are able to tie off blood vessels so that they can see more clearly, instead of blindly cutting and ripping. Better isolation and control of blood vessels also means that there is less drastic blood loss during the operation. Before Walsh's improvements, blood transfusions were common during radical prostatectomies. Today, transfusions are often unnecessary. The modern radical prostatectomy is less traumatic compared to what it was before the anatomic approach was developed, but it still remains major surgery.

Myth Busting Quiz

1) If you remove the entire prostate and all the cancer that can be seen within it, prostate cancer is definitely cured. Yes or no?

2) Having prostate cancer is always worse than having prostate cancer surgery. Yes or no?

3) Some men who undergo the nerve-sparing radial prostatectomy will have normal sexual function afterwards. Yes or no?

4) Controlled studies have shown the radical prostatectomy to extend life. Yes or no?

5) Randomized controlled studies have proven the radical prostatectomy to extend survival and to be better than other treatments for prostate cancer. Yes or no?

The answer is no for every question. Read on to understand why.

The Operation

To do the anatomic approach to the radical prostatectomy, the man's lower abdomen is sliced open; arteries and veins are found, and they are severed and tied off to gain "control" of the operating field, which means stopping the bleeding enough so that the surgeon can proceed to isolate and remove the prostate. Once tied off, however, you do not get these arteries and veins back.

With Walsh's technique, surgeons can sometimes find the two nerve trunks that pass along the outside of the prostate, which innervate *some* of the male sexual structures. They have the option of sparing these nerves, or widely excising them if cancer may be escaping along them. Other urologists began using the term "nerve-sparing" to describe saving the two nerve trunks around the prostate. Today, Walsh's method of doing the radical prostatectomy is often called nerve-sparing when one or both nerve trunks are saved instead of severed.

Unfortunately, the term nerve-sparing is often used in very misleading fashion. Men have reported the following type of conversation to me:

"You need surgery," the urologist says.

"What about impotence?"

"We'll spare the nerves."

I think many men come away from such conversations with the wrong impression about what nerve-sparing actually means. Recently a man said to me, "I'm impotent after surgery, but it can't be the nerves, they were spared." As we will see, while two nerve trunks can be spared, most nerves are cut.

Walsh's anatomic approach to the radical prostatectomy is largely about blood control, while nerve sparing is an entirely separate issue. Since the two new techniques are sometimes done together they are often confused.

Dr. Walsh found that the two nerve trunks that go around the prostate could be spared, and they are important to penile sensation, but unfortunately, usually at least eight nerve branches are cut. These branches are vital to getting and maintaining a full erection, frequent erections, and in many cases to getting an erection at all. Somehow men don't get the picture that so many nerves are cut and removed during an RP, even when nerve-sparing is done.

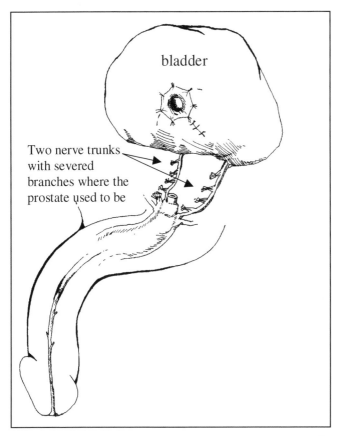

Figure 17. Even when "bilateral nerve-sparing" is done, eight nerves are still cut, as well as the veins and arteries that go with them. (Artist: Jun Macam)

How often are both nerve trunks spared? Not as often as you might think. Urologists often sacrifice the nerve trunk on the side where the cancer is. They usually cut it and excise widely around it in an attempt to get all the cancer. In effect, it's not unusual for nine out of 10 nerves to be severed—one of the two nerve trunks is cut and eight nerve branches are cut. In reality, the "nerve-sparing" radical prostatectomy is not very "nerve-sparing."

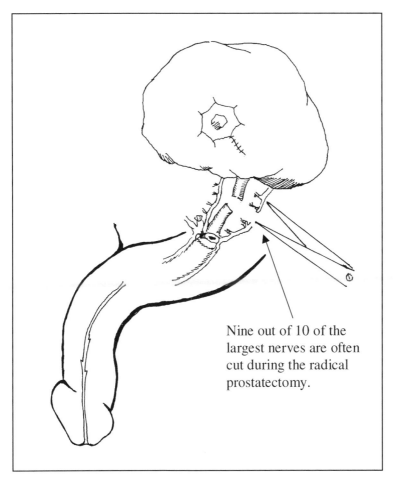

Nine out of 10 of the largest nerves are often cut during the radical prostatectomy.

Figure 18. Eight Nerve branches are cut, and about half the time, one nerve branch is cut during a typical radical prostatectomy. (Artist: Jun Macam)

Along with the eight nerve branches and one nerve trunk, all the arteries and veins that travel with these nerves are also severed. It's no wonder that the penis, which requires nerves, arteries, and veins to function, can never be expected to be the same after a radical prostatectomy.

The use of the term nerve-sparing as applied to the radical prostatectomy is largely inappropriate. No one makes the point more strongly that urologist Patrick Walsh:

> "Firstly, let me dispel the notion of 'nerve-sparing radical prostatectomy.' Many people use that term when referring to the operation that I developed. However, this terminology is inaccurate. I refer to this operation as an 'Anatomical Approach to Radical Prostatectomy.' This operation has been perfected over the past 15 years and essentially involves 3 steps: (1) accurate control of bleeding to provide a relatively bloodless field; (2) intraoperative assessment of the extent of tumor; and (3) preservation or wide excision of the nerves where necessary.
>
> "Prior to the advent of this procedure, the nerves were never excised—they were just cut and left in place. With the development of an anatomical approach to radical prostatectomy, it is now possible to preserve the nerves where feasible or excise them widely where necessary to provide an adequate surgical margin . . . . In actuality, both neurovascular bundles are spared in only 58 percent of patients."[144]

---

[144] Walsh, Patrick C: Reply to Article by Stamey on Prostate Cancer. *Oncolink.* September 1, 1994. Available at: http://oncolink.upenn.edu/disease/prostate/treatment/walsh.html. Quoted with signed, written permission.

Cancer Control

If the surgeon can really do a better job with the new improved radical prostatectomy, he should get all of the prostate cancer out more often than with the old, "1904-style operation." When the removed prostate is taken out, there should be fewer instances where the margins are positive for cancer. When positive margins occur it means that some cancer has been left behind.

The anatomic radical prostatectomy with nerve sparing may be a "better" operation in some regards, but it is not unquestionably the advance in cancer control that many would like to believe. The nerve sparing approach can actually make the operation more likely to fail because cancer is more likely to be left behind along the nerves that are spared.

Prostate cancer seems to enjoy spreading along the paths of nerves. Thus there is a debate about whether positive margins for cancer are more likely to occur with nerve sparing surgery than with the old radical prostatectomy in which the nerves were not spared. It's a controversy that has not been satisfactorily resolved.

Most men don't realize that the two nerve trunks for erection are enclosed in a sheath called the periprostatic fossa that adheres to the prostate. This sheath must be incised and the nerves dissected away from the prostate to save them. Many prostate cancers are thought to escape the prostate by following along these nerves—so leaving them may leave cancer. Dr. Walsh, when first doing his new technique of radical prostatectomy, had perhaps the highest rate of positive surgical margins ever published, until he modified his operation to include wide excision of the nerve trunks in many cases. And wide excision of the nerves removes the sparing of sexual function advantage for which many men are choosing the modern version of surgery in the first place.

Part of the problem is that the surgeon cannot see micro-metastases that are escaping the prostate. It only takes a few escaping prostate cancer cells to spread the disease. For this reason, urologists don't know with certainty when to spare the nerves, versus when to widely excise the nerves.

The Radical Prostatectomy and Your Penis

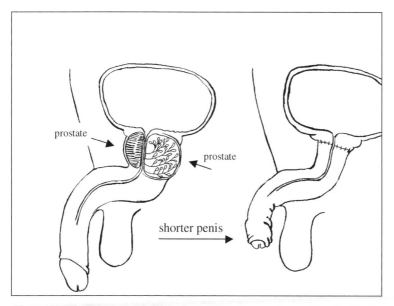

Figure 19. The prostate is still present on the left. On the right, after the radical prostatectomy, the penis is pulled up and sutured to the bladder. The length of penis extending out of the body is reduced, and the circumcised man may now appear to be uncircumcised. (Artist: Jun Macam)

Many men will notice a shorter penis immediately after radical surgery. The immediate decrease in size is due to the penis being pulled up into the pelvis. The radical prostatectomy removes the prostate and thus the penis is usually pulled up into the body to be attached to the bladder. The body has a wonderful ability to stretch after surgery, but not to the full extent of the one to two inches lost when the prostate is taken out. Some men will complain of losing only a few millimeters; others will complain of losing so much that, even though they are circumcised, they appear to have foreskin again; the penis has been drawn up that far. It's not uncommon for men to say that they lost an inch in length. Men will also complain about shortening and changing of the angle of their penises. One man complains that if he is not careful when he sits on the toilet, the angle of his shorter penis causes his urine to shoot out under the lid of the toilet and onto the floor.

This shortening is only the beginning of the damage. Men will also note additional shrinkage of their penises over time, due to nerves, arteries, and veins that nourish the penis being cut during the RP. Once the penis is without its blood supply and nerves it withers away. Doctors say that it *atrophies.*

There is a 100 percent risk of a smaller penis after the radical prostatectomy, and there is a 100 percent rate of sexual dysfunction after the radical prostatectomy. Dr. Walsh and his colleagues published this statement:

> "When potent patients were asked to estimate the quality of erection compared to preoperative status, patients stated that it averaged 79% of preoperative status (range 60 to 95%)."[145]

Note the range of Dr. Walsh's study. No man in the study, who could get an erection, achieved an erection after the RP that was as good as before surgery.

One study presented at the 1998 American Urological Association Convention examined the penises of 90 men who had undergone nerve sparing radical prostatectomy. Doctors measured both the flaccid state and the erect state

---

[145] Walsh, Patrick C, Alan W. Partin and Jonathan I. Epstein: Cancer Control and Quality of Life Following Anatomical Radical Retropubic Prostatectomy: Results at 10 years. *Journal of Urology.* November 1994;152(5 Pt 2):1831-1836. Quoted with signed, written permission.

(although the men had to be given shots into their penises to achieve an erect state). The authors reported that there was a 9 percent decrease in flaccid and erect length, and a 7 percent decrease in flaccid and erect circumference, after radical prostatectomy at an average follow-up time of 7 months. The lost of length and girth resulted in a *27 percent loss in volume* of the penis.[146]

Sexual Dysfunction

I asked twenty-one men who had a nerve-sparing radical prostatectomy if they suffered from any of the following:

1) Loss of sensation in the penis (penis feels dead)
2) A cold penis
3) A penis that feels shriveled, as if coming out of a cold swimming pool
4) Fewer erections than before radical prostatectomy
5) Erections that are only partial at best
6) Difficulty achieving orgasm

Some men answered all the questions, and others answered some of them.

- Four of 15 men (27 percent) noted a loss of sensation to the penis
- Four of 16 men (25 percent) noted a cold penis after RP
- Eight of 14 men (57 percent) noted that their penis had shriveled

---

[146] McCullough AR, and Lepor H: The loss of penile length and circumference in impotent men after nerve sparing radical prostatectomy. *Journal of Urology.* 1998;159(5)Supplement:98. Abstract number 376 presented at the 1998 AUA convention. Available at http://www.auanet.org/annualmeet98/abstracts/AUA98_03750.html.

- Eighteen of 18 (100 percent) noted fewer erections than before; nine of these 18 added that they were unable to achieve any erections at all
- Twenty of 20 (100 percent) noted only partial erections at best; nine of these twenty were unable to realize an erection at all
- Eleven of 15 (73 percent) reported difficulty achieving orgasm, using terms like "only a shadow," "possible," "have them but different," "some pain," and "not sure it happens," to describe orgasms after a radical prostatectomy.

What does such a survey mean? First, the radical prostatectomy is devastating to male sexual function. Second, it only takes a small sample size to reveal side effects that occur after the radical prostatectomy, which have never been mentioned in the medical literature and that men were not warned about before surgery.

It's clear that the radical prostatectomy means fewer erections and partial erections at best. I always tell men that there is a 100 percent rate of sexual dysfunction after the radical prostatectomy, meaning that men after RP get far fewer erections or no erections at all, and that they get smaller "less quality" erections.

It gets worse. In addition to lousy or no erections, men have no semen to ejaculate at orgasm. Orgasm can never be the same after radical prostatectomy, because the prostate and seminal vesicles, which contract during orgasm, are gone. Forever after the radical prostatectomy, men will have dry climaxes if they are able to achieve erection and climax at all.

The demonstration of how important the nerves sacrificed during the radical prostatectomy are has been elegantly demonstrated in an animal study. Dr. Peter Chan and his colleagues documented what many of us have already concluded from the experiences of men post-RP, namely that the branches of the nerves that are cut during the radical prostatectomy are vital for getting normal, completely rigid, erections. Chan's animal model showed that when these nerve branches are cut, softer, smaller, erections occur even with chemically induced erections.[147]

Sexual Dysfunction Statistics

Impotence statistics after radical prostatectomy are very distorted. In the medical literature, one of the ways that urologists follow up on sexual function after the RP is to ask men if they have had *one* (emphasis on one) erection hard enough to penetrate a vagina in the last 4 weeks. If men achieved one such erection within the 4-week period they are said to be potent in such studies.

This is a horrible way to be measuring sexual potency, although it's a favorable way to measure it for someone who wants to promote surgery. No man will have as good sexual function after RP as before the surgery; it's anatomically impossible. The existing data makes this incontrovertibly clear, yet this data is not being disseminated to men as loudly as it should be.

I watched a urologist on television say, "Many men will have normal sexual function after prostate surgery," when talking about the radical prostatectomy. Such a statement is misleading. Sexual function post-RP is normal only if you consider smaller, less frequent, semi-hard erections to be normal—not to mention sterility, poor orgasms, and decreased libido. There's nothing normal about sex after a radical prostatectomy.

The new wonder drug for erectile dysfunction, Viagra, has been a disappointment for men after radical prostatectomy. Supposedly, about 40 percent of men after radical prostatectomy, especially if they have bilateral nerve sparing and are young, can achieve erections on Viagra. The

---

[147] Chan PT, Philippe E. Spiess, Peter Zvara, Scott L. Merlin, Ste'phane B. Dion, and Gerald B. Brock: Preservation of penile erectile function post-prostatectomy in rat using a micro-surgical procedure with sparing of the antero-lateral branches of the cavernous nerves.

converse is that for many men after RP, Viagra only gives them a fluffier penis without any hardness.

During the radical prostatectomy, some of the blood supply to the pelvic area is severed in order to see better during the operation, and when the urologist removes the prostate many important structures, such as veins, arteries, and nerves are severed. So how well can Viagra, Cialis, or Levitra work?

Many men post radical prostatectomy have been very disappointed and describe getting only larger, flaccid, penises after Viagra. A recent paper suggests that Viagra never works for men who do not have a nerve-sparing radical prostatectomy and even in those who have a unilateral nerve-sparing procedure it may not work.[148] Since most men are getting unilateral nerve-sparing procedures it seems doubtful that Viagra will be helpful for men after an RP unless they have a bilateral nerve sparing procedure, and then the response may well be significantly less than 100 percent.

The most important thing is not to have a radical prostatectomy with the belief that Viagra will give you normal erections after the operation. Based on the currently available data, it probably won't.

---

[148] Zippe CD, Kedia AW, Kedia K, Nelson DR, and Agarwal A: Treatment of erectile dysfunction after radical prostatectomy with sildenafil citrate (Viagra). UROLOGY. 1998;52(6):963-966.

Impotence After the Radical Prostatectomy

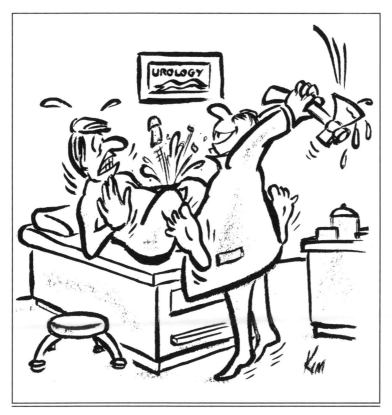

Figure 20. "I wanted a radical prostatectomy, not my penis cut off!" (Artist: Mike Kim)

Introduction

At age 60, John, who had worked hard all his life, was looking forward to retirement. He had made a fortune and planned on traveling the world with his wife, with whom he was still very much in love. He was also looking forward to more frequent sex with her now that the kids were out of the house.

Before leaving on the trip, John visited his hometown doctor for a physical. His doctor did a digital rectal exam (DRE), which was normal. The doctor also ordered a prostate specific antigen (PSA) blood test as a screen for prostate cancer.

John's PSA level was found to be elevated, indicating that cancer might be present. John was stunned; he had no symptoms whatsoever. He felt fine!

John was referred to a urologist. The urologist performed a biopsy and prostate cancer was present in one of John's biopsy specimens.

A few weeks later, John underwent a radical prostatectomy. After a bumpy four weeks of recovery, John soon realized that he would never be the same. He was impotent. He had to wear a diaper because he leaked urine all the time. He took several showers a day in a futile effort to keep the smell of urine off himself. He couldn't make love to his wife after the surgery, and eventually realized he would never have an erection again.

His leaking urine kept him from going out for breakfast every morning as he used to do, or from visiting his grandchildren. He could do neither without staining his clothes with urine. The stench of his own urine was always burning his nostrils.

The more he read about prostate cancer, the more John was sure that he had been terribly misinformed about the quality of life he could expect after the operation. He wondered if with his low PSA level and low Gleason score, he might have not lived 10 years without any symptoms from his prostate cancer—long enough to fulfill all his retirement dreams. He was stressed beyond belief by the results of his radical prostatectomy. John died a bitter man—of a heart attack—two years after his surgery.

Like many men, John underwent the radical prostatectomy without knowing what to expect with respect to his sexuality. All men should expect a *100 percent rate of sexual dysfunction.* They will be infertile, will not have semen, orgasm will not be the same, and they will suffer smaller penises; they are also more likely to be impotent than not. The statistics on impotence after the radical prostatectomy vary from 10 percent to 90 percent, one urologist even telling me 100 percent, but most of the studies reporting lower rates of impotence are seriously flawed studies. The lowest impotency rates are seen in studies that select out men who are less than 50 years old and have both nerve trunks spared at surgery—I question whether such young men should have had surgery in the first place. Most men operated on are in their 60s and 70s, with arguably, less to lose, but I think no man should lose his sexuality.

Studies showing the highest rates of impotence tend to be ones based upon survey questions that delve deeply into details about sexual performance, and are "patient driven." One might reasonably expect that scientists who are not urologists would present the most unbiased data as urologists have an obvious economic-based conflict of interest in presenting such information.

What does potent mean? According to Thomas Stamey, MD, at one point in time, most sexual follow-up surveys were based on the question: "Have you had successful intercourse with vaginal penetration at least once in the past year?" This question was—inadvertently or not—heavily skewed to support claims of potency after RP. More recent studies ask if one erection sufficient for intercourse has occurred in the last four weeks.

Why four weeks? Why not ask about an erection capable of intercourse in the last 24 hours, or the last one-week? Few sexually active men would consider one erection every 4 weeks to be the definition of virility.

It's no wonder that studies done by urologists and patient oriented surveys often report drastically different numbers. Results depend on how you define impotence or its opposite, potency. Fortunately, more and more studies are defining potency as the ability to have an unassisted erection sufficient for vaginal penetration and orgasm on a regular basis. Now we need to pin down "regular basis." The truth is that men should be able to have erections sufficient for sexual intercourse on a daily basis, or twice daily basis, almost regardless of their age. My other books, *The Prostatitis Syndromes* and *Prostatitis and BPH*, explain how men can keep their prostates clean of debris and small in size throughout their lives, thus preserving life-long sexual function.

The Math of Sexual Potency

I want to explain why the potency statistics after RP are statistical lies. Suppose one hundred men can achieve at least one erection per day (use your own number if you wish). These men can achieve a total of 36,500 erections per year. Now assume that these same 100 potent men all undergo radical prostatectomy.

Suppose that after the surgery, only 15 of the men get an erection hard enough for intercourse once a month (this is one real-world scenario). This means that the number of possible erections is down in our group of men from 36,500 per year to only 180 erections per year. That's a 99 percent reduction in erections!

In the best situation, if all our men are under fifty and have both of their nerve trunks spared, according to one study, 90 percent of them will get a serviceable erection once every four weeks. And, if only once a month, this gives our men 1,300 usable erections per year, instead of 36,500. That's a 96 percent decline in the number of erections that can be achieved! Why aren't potency statistics presented this way?

I've just shown you that how you define potency makes an incredible difference. With the last example, you could either say that 90 percent of the men were potent after RP or that there was a 96 percent decline in number of erections the men could obtain. Which is more truthful?

Sex after the RP ultimately ends on a tragic note. The radical prostatectomy creates shorter, less serviceable penises, and poor quality erections, if erections are achieved at all. Post-RP men are sterile since they don't ejaculate any semen.

Post-RP men are forced to go to extremes to have sex, needing more direct stimulation of the penis, greater use of pornography, penile vacuum pumps, shots of vasoactive drugs into their penises, or other aids to have sex. Viagra has not been an overwhelming success in men after radical prostatectomy. Too many nerves, arteries, and veins have been destroyed by the typical RP for it to have the kind of effectiveness it has in men who are anatomically intact. Some post-RP men leak urine when they try to have sex after their RP, another situation that reduces sexual activity. In fact, many things happen post-RP that invariably affect sex or the sex drive. One seldom mentioned problem is that when the prostate is removed so is all the dihydrotestosterone (DHT), a powerful male sex hormone. The real tragedy may not be the loss of sex, but that in all the manipulations to preserve sex, what has clearly been lost is the ability to make love—at least spontaneously.

One man who underwent RP gives this advice:

"Most of all, I would try very hard to hold on to my prostate—once it is removed, it is gone forever. Who knows, they may come up with a magic bullet tomorrow—but if your prostate is gone, it won't do you any good. Once the prostate is gone, you will probably be impotent, unable to have a normal erection. Even if you are one of the lucky few who are still able to have an erection, sex will never be the same—you will have no ejaculate and since the prostate is actively involved in orgasm by squeezing down to force the ejaculate out, you will be missing a large part of the pleasure of an orgasm. I am one of the unlucky many who is impotent—have to use a vacuum device or stick my penis with a needle in order to have an erection. You may also have incontinence— some have it for the rest of their life. I had a radical prostatectomy 5 years ago. I still have an incontinence problem. I would give any amount of money to have my prostate back."[149]

[149] Aubrey Pilgram. *A Revolutionary Approach to Prostate Cancer.* Sterling House 1998. With permission.

Sexual Function Inventory

One tool that helps men decide about surgery is the sexual function inventory shown below.[150] Every man contemplating radical prostatectomy should be given this fourteen-question sexual function inventory prior to surgery as well as afterwards. Every man contemplating an RP should be started on Viagra, Cialis, or Levitra, and take the inventory again, so that he knows what he has to lose by surgery.

And, an expanded inventory should be the basis for a large-scale study delineating exactly what happens to men's sex lives after the radical prostatectomy. We should know exactly which symptoms of sexual dysfunction occur post-RP and how often, but we don't, despite tens of thousands of radical prostatectomies being done every year.

1.   Before surgery, were you able to have an adequate erection for intercourse?
        Yes_____   No_____
2. How rigid was your erection prior to therapy?
        No rigidity_____   Some rigidity_____   Excellent rigidity_____
3.   Prior to surgery, was your erection rigid enough to penetrate?
        Never_____   Sometimes_____   Always_____

---

[150] Chaikin, David C, Gregory A. Broderick, Terrence R. Malloy, S. Bruce Malkowicz, Richard Whittington, and Alan J. Wein: Erectile Dysfunction Following Minimally Invasive Treatments for Prostate Cancer. UROLOGY. 1996; vol. 48: pages 100-104. Reprinted with signed, written permission from Elsevier Science.

4. Prior to surgery, did your erection last long enough to have an orgasm?

Never_____   Sometimes_____   Always_____

5. Prior to surgery, how was your sexual drive?

Poor_____   Good_____   Very good_____

6. Prior to surgery, would viewing sexually erotic materials or masturbation produce an erection?

No_____   Sometimes_____   Always_____

7. Prior to surgery, how was the sensitivity (feeling) of your penis?

Decreased_____   Adequate_____   Very good_____

8.   In the last 4 weeks, have you been able to have an adequate erection for intercourse?

Yes_____   No_____

9. Compared to before surgery, how rigid are your erections?

No rigidity_____   Decreased rigidity_____   No change_____

10.   Since surgery, has your erection been rigid enough for penetration?

Never_____   Less often than before surgery_____ No change_____

11.   Since surgery, does your erection last long enough to reach orgasm?

Never_____   Less often than before surgery_____ No change_____

12.   Since surgery, how has your sexual drive been?

Worse_____   No change_____   Better_____

13.   Since surgery, does viewing sexually explicit materials or masturbation produce erection?

Never_____   Less often than before surgery_____ No change_____

14.   Since surgery, how is the sensitivity (feeling) of your penis?

Decreased_____   No change_____   Increased_____

Men Lie about Sex

Men lie about sex all the time. I sometimes monitor support groups, Internet mailing lists, and a newsgroup on prostate cancer and am often amazed at the lies men tell themselves.

Some men claim to have normal sexual function after the radical prostatectomy. They are redefining normal to suit their disability. It's anatomically impossible to have normal sexual function after the radical prostatectomy. Sure, the rare man, usually young, with bilateral nerve sparing, with a small cancer, who shouldn't have had surgery in the first place in my opinion, will claim to do well sexually. But no man will ever return to normal. Men delude themselves by rationalizing that having no semen, having smaller penises, or having sex less often is somehow normal. One man insisted on an Internet list that his penis did not decrease in size after the RP. He also admitted to using a vacuum erection device. I did not point out the obvious—damage occurred or such manipulations would not be needed.

Urologists have joined in the deception by publishing ridiculous studies in which they insert a catheter and pull the penis back out and measure it, which of course would make the length appear to be normal again. Or they do measurements after stretching the penis and then claim its length is still normal. Both these techniques attempt to cover up that the radical prostatectomy pulls the penis up inside the body and causes it to atrophy.

In addition, a few men will claim to have normal or better orgasms after the radical prostatectomy. I believe this happens only in a few men who had diseased prostates and seminal vesicles before surgery, which dragged down their orgasms to a lower level. Their prostates were probably swollen with prostatitis, BPH, and prostate cancer before surgery. Getting rid of their diseased organs allows their pelvic muscles to contract during orgasm without as much resistance. However, urologists should not let men's prostates and seminal vesicles become so diseased before intervening. In any event, dry orgasms, without the contractions of the prostate and seminal vesicles, are not normal.

After the radical prostatectomy do not expect to make spontaneous love again. Expect to use drugs, injections, and devices to have sex, if you can have sex at all.

The Radical Prostatectomy and Incontinence

Imagine leaking urine every time you stand up. Imagine dribbling urine down your legs every time you take a step. Imagine your groin being raw and moist with the sickly smell of urine. Imagine trying to have sex with a semi-functional erection and leaking urine all over yourself and your sex partner. Imagine waking up in your own urine every morning. Imagine having to know where the restroom is at all times; you can hold your urine for 100 feet but you can't hold it long enough to drive home.

Incontinence is a very serious side effect when it comes to quality of life. Even having to wear one pad per day can be devastating.

Men have three urinary sphincters in my opinion: one at the top of the prostate, the prostate itself, and one at the bottom of the prostate (Urologists don't count the prostate itself as a sphincter, which I do). The radical prostatectomy removes the top urinary sphincter and the prostate. This leaves only one urinary sphincter behind, and it is often damaged by the operation.

The reported incontinence rate after the radical prostatectomy varies widely from study to study. One view is that all men are incontinent after radical prostatectomy; it's just a matter of how you define it. At the other extreme are the urologists who claim that surgical technique is so improved that most men are completely dry even when stressed by coughing, straining, or lifting.

Some studies define the man who drips a couple of drops a day as being continent. Others say such men are incontinent. The best studies available are those that define incontinence with greatest specificity, enumerating exactly the number of pads used to soak up urine, indicating if any dripping of urine occurs, and under what circumstances.

Men who leak urine when they cough or strain are "stress incontinent," but many studies don't even ask about this. The man who was once continent but now never puts any strain on his abdominal muscles so that he will not leak urine has not come through the operation with complete urinary continence. He's dancing on eggshells to stay continent, instead of leading an active life.

The urological literature often announces low rates of incontinence while independent sources publish higher rates of incontinence. It's likely that surveys of patients are more accurate than reports by urologists, which are often overly optimistic.

The Medicare incontinence study

In a study that I know to have been done by careful researchers, 32 percent of post-radical prostatectomy men ended up wearing pads or a clamp on their penis to deal with urine leakage.[151] When those who did at least some dripping are factored in, 47 percent of the Medicare patients surveyed dripped urine on a daily basis after their radical prostatectomy.

Harvard Incontinence study

One prospective and thorough study on post-RP incontinence was done at Harvard. Of 125 men studied, two years after surgery 15 percent described themselves as "leaking urine a lot." Altogether 42 percent of men were

---

[151] Fowler, Floyd J. Jr., Michael J. Barry, Grace Lu-Yao, John H. Wasson, and Lin Bin; Outcomes of External-Bean Radiation Therapy for Prostate Cancer: A Study of Medicare Beneficiaries in Three Surveillance, Epidemiology, and End Results Areas. *Journal of Clinical Oncology.* 1996:14(8):2258-2265.

wearing pads in their underwear to soak up urine two years after surgery.[152]

The Study by the American College of Surgeons

A study headed by the American College of Surgeons of 2,122 men with a PSA over 4, and younger than 75 when the radical prostatectomy was done, found that 3.6 percent of the men were totally incontinent, 4.1 percent of the men wore more than 2 pads daily to soak up leaking urine, 11.2 percent of the men wore 2 pads or less per day, and 23 percent dripped occasionally but did not wear pads. Overall, 42 percent of the men were leaking in some fashion while 58 percent were dry. [153]

Dr. Patrick Walsh's Study

Urologist Patrick Walsh announced on the Internet the results of his 10-year study of incontinence among his first 500 radical prostatectomy patients. The men were operated on between 1982 and 1988. According to his Internet announcement, 92 percent of his first 500 patients are dry, while 8 percent either wear pads or have stress incontinence.[154]

---

[152] JA Talcott, P Rieker, KJ Propert, J Clark, P Kantoff, Dana Farber Cancer Institute; C Beard, I Kaplan, Joint Center for Radiation Therapy; K. Loughlin, J Richie, Brigham and Women's Hospital; and K Wishnow, New England Deaconess Hospital: Long-Term Complications of Treatment for early Prostate Cancer: 2-Year follow up in a prospective, multi-institutional outcomes study, Abstract No. 644, Proceedings of Asco Vol. 15, March 1996, *Genitourinary Tract Cancer*.

[153] Murphy, Gerald P., Curtis Mettlin, Herman Menck, David P. Winchester and Anna Marie Davidson: National Patterns of Prostate Cancer Treatment by Radical Prostatectomy: Results of a Survey by the American College of Surgeons Commission on Cancer, *Journal of Urology*. November 1994: Vol. 152, 1817-1819.

[154] Walsh, Patrick C. Reply to Article by Stamey on Prostate Cancer. 1994. Available at http://cancer.med.upenn.edu/disease/prostate/treatment/walsh.html.

Why are Walsh's numbers so much better than everyone else's? One possible reason could be that he performs the operation better than anyone else. He has a lot of fans that think that this is true. Of course if some urologists are achieving these high levels of continence, then an awful lot of urologists would have to be leaving most of their patients incontinent most of the time, to achieve the average rates of incontinence that other studies are reporting.

Lastly, I do not want to leave you with the impression that sexual dysfunction and incontinence are the only side effects of the radical prostatectomy. There is a huge laundry list of side effects ranging from death on the operating table to chronic constipation to lymph node damage. Time doesn't allow me to list all the side effects that men have suffered from the radical prostatectomy, and the more men that I interview, the more side effects I uncover.

The Radical Prostatectomy and Quality of Life

Doctors and patients are often not on the same page when it comes to side effects.

> ". . . do doctors have any understanding of how their patients actually live in the real world?"[155]

> "It is a well-known fact that doctors experience complications differently from patients."[156]

> "Unfortunately, I will never fully recover from the surgery. Since surgery I have been sexually impotent, and I continue to have daily physical symptoms such as radiating pain in my lower back and legs; abdominal and joint pain and various other disconcerting pains which occur randomly in my muscles and throughout my body; I am not fully continent; I fatigue easily; and last, but certainly not least,

---

[155] Korda, Michael. *Man to Man: Surviving Prostate Cancer.* New York: Random House.1996, p. 171. Quoted with signed, written permission.

[156] Altwein J, Ekman P, Barry M, Biermann C, Carlsson P, Fossa S, Kiebert G, Kuchler T, McLeod D, Porter A, and Steineck G: How is Quality of Life in Prostate Cancer Patients Influenced by Modern Treatment? The Wallenberg Symposium. UROLOGY. 1997;49(suppl4a):66-76. Reprinted from Urology. Copyright 1997. Quoted with signed, written permission from Elsevier Science.

the cancer continued to grow, necessitating further treatment."[157]

Doctors are often able to ignore side effects far more easily than the men who have to live with them. And, the perception of side effects changes over time as men are forced to live with them. One study found that immediately after having a radical prostatectomy most patients would undergo the surgery again, but after living with incontinence for five years over half the men regretted the operation and, if they could go back in time, would not have it again.[158]

Modeling Studies

A study published in the *Journal of the American Medical Association* (JAMA) in 1993 was a landmark because researchers finally took into account the fact that the quality of life goes down significantly—even drastically—in men who undergo a radical prostatectomy.[159] The authors created a computer model to see how much benefit there would be from having a radical prostatectomy, when taking into account the side effects and as many other variables as they could, including the fact that most prostate cancer patients die from other causes (competing mortality) than prostate cancer. They started by building in some pretty generous assumptions in favor of the radical prostatectomy. Nonetheless, they came to some pretty startling conclusions. They created six scenarios by varying

---

[157] Lewis, James: *New Guidelines for Surviving Prostate Cancer.* New York: Health Education Literary Publisher 1997. Page 73. Quoted with signed, written permission.

[158] Herr HW: Quality of life of incontinent men after radical prostatectomy. *Journal of Urology.* 1994;151:652-654.

[159] Fleming C, Wasson JH, Albertsen PC, Barry MJ, Wennberg JE, for the Prostate Patient Outcomes Research Team: A decision analysis of alternative treatment strategies for clinically localized prostate cancer. JAMA, 1993;269:2650-2658.

the estimated efficacy rates of the radical prostatectomy and by varying the presumed metastatic rate of prostate cancer. In three of the six scenarios, undergoing radical prostatectomy did not give men any increase in "quality of life" years at all. In the three scenarios—making more favorable assumptions—the highest quality of life benefit was 3.4 years for the RP, but in every situation in which the RP showed a benefit, external beam radiation therapy provided more benefit.

The authors concluded that for many men, watchful waiting was a reasonable alternative to radical prostatectomy. Men who don't have the opportunity to read the medical literature would be surprised by the extraordinary "cat fight" that this study caused. Urologists wrote to JAMA and bitterly defended their operation saying that the modeling study was of "limited relevance," and calling it "ghastly." The authors replied that there was little credible evidence that the radical prostatectomy generally worked, even when using optimistic assumptions, pointing out that the history of medicine is replete with drastic treatments that were enthusiastically promoted before controlled studies showed them to be of no benefit.

The most bizarre turn to the story is that the authors were asked to provide their model's data for a critique, which they did. Based on their data, other authors created a new model, which perhaps not surprisingly, showed that under better assumptions the radical prostatectomy had an increase in quality-adjusted life years for low-grade prostate cancer of 1.81 years, for medium-grade prostate cancer of 2.94 years, and for high-grade cancer of 2.34 years.[160] The new model was published in the *Journal of Urology*, not JAMA, and a commentary by the original authors was not published simultaneously with the results of the new model as would have been appropriate.

---

[160] Beck JR, Kattan MW, and Miles BJ: A Critique of the Decision Analysis for Clinically Localized Prostate Cancer. *Journal of Urology*. 1994;152:1894-1899

Another modeling study appeared in JAMA and it suggested that any benefit of the radical prostatectomy was more than offset by the harm that the radical prostatectomy does to men.[161]

Quality of Life

One of the problems with the radical prostatectomy is that study after study reports results in a biased fashion, while totally ignoring quality of life issues from the patients' point of view. Survival and quality of life must both be considered. For many men, quality of life is paramount. A study commissioned by Us TOO International found that men consider quality of life most important, followed by length of life. These men said that 30 percent of the time their doctor did not discuss how prostate cancer treatment would affect their quality of life.[162]

At the heart of the controversy is the surgeon's built-in bias for performing surgery. Some question whether it's really in the patients' best interests that the people who benefit the most, financially and emotionally, from the operation are almost exclusively in charge of collecting and evaluating the data determining whether or not the operation works, or has side effects. How can the urologist, who may get $8,000 for doing a radical prostatectomy, and who went into surgery because he likes to operate, be the person to most objectively assess his most lucrative operation?

---

[161] Krahn MD, Mahoney JE, Eckman MH, Trachtenberg J, Pauker SG, Detsky AS: Screening for Prostate Cancer: A Decision Analytic View. *Journal of the American Medical Association.* 1994;272(10):773-780.

[162] Henry A. Porterfield, Chair/CEO of Us TOO International, "Introduction from the Chairman," *Louis Harris & Associates Survey, Perspectives on Prostate Cancer Treatment: Awareness, Attitudes and Relationships—A Study of Patients and Urologists.* 1995. Us TOO International, Inc. Prostate Cancer Support Groups. Available at http://www.ustoo.com/louis.html. Quoted with signed, written permission by Hank P. and Louis Harris and Associates.

In his book, *Man to Man: Surviving Prostate Cancer*, Michael Korda relates that:

> ". . . a lot of patients feel hustled into the operating room unnecessarily, in the doctor's interests rather than their own . . . it certainly *does* matter that a surgeon's instinctive bias is, naturally, toward cutting."[163]

---

[163] Michael Korda. *Man to Man Surviving Prostate Cancer.* New York: Vintage Books: A Division of Random House, Inc. 1997. Page 39. Copyright 1996, 1997 by Success Research Corporation. Quoted with signed, written permission.

Does the Radical Prostatectomy Work?

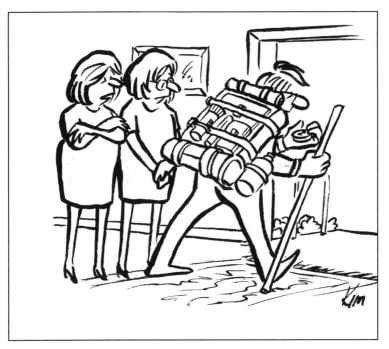

Figure 21. "He's off to find a urologist who operates based only on randomized controlled trials. He may be gone for the rest of our lives!" (Artist: Mike Kim)

Introduction

At a prostate cancer support group, I asked a urologist, "What's the cure rate for the radical prostatectomy?"

"It's 80 percent," he said.

I also asked some of the men who had underwent radical prostatectomy what they had been told the cure rate was. I heard 88 percent from one man and 95 percent from another.

I read a passage in which a urologist stated the radical prostatectomy had the highest cure rate for prostate cancer ever reported.

I've been to several conferences for the lay public where urologists speak. Often lecturing urologists will tell the audience that the radical prostatectomy has a cure rate in the range of 80 percent or better for prostate cancer.

Such statements are lies.

According to the scientific information we have today, if you select out men as they are selected out for radical prostatectomy, and don't do surgery, the majority of them will not die from prostate cancer. So, it's impossible to have a cure rate of 80 – 95 percent when most of the men being operated on don't need curing in the first place! Urologists incorrectly and shamelessly include needless surgery as success.

A Prospective Study in JAMA by Jan-Erik Johansson et al.

The Journal of the American Medical Association published a remarkable study in 1997. It was called "Fifteen-Year Survival in Prostate Cancer: A Prospective, Population-Based Study in Sweden."[164] It was a well-done study and demonstrated how difficult it is to show that the radical prostatectomy, or any other local therapy, benefits patients. It found a 15-year survival rate of 81 percent for 223 patients with watchful waiting, and a 15-year survival rate of 81 percent for 77 men who had local therapy, either by radiation (75 patients) or by radical prostatectomy (2 patients).

---

[164] Jan-Erik Johansson, Lars Holmberg, Sara Johannson, Reinhold Bergström, and Hans-Olov Adami: Fifteen Year Survival in Prostate Cancer: A Prospective, Population-Based Study in Sweden. JAMA. 1997;277(6):467-471.

The watchful waiting aspect of the study set a benchmark with respect to therapies for prostate cancer. It demonstrated that 81 percent of the prostate cancer patients studied didn't require treatment to achieve 15-year survival.

Also in 1997, the same year Dr. Johansson's study was published, he told me that he had never taken the PSA test. Fifty-two years old at the time, it was his view that neither the radical prostatectomy nor any other therapy was scientifically proven to work for prostate cancer. He told me that he would himself deal with prostate cancer, if he ever came down with it, only if symptoms occurred. In 2003, at the age of 57, he emailed me and repeated that if he had symptoms, he would take the PSA test.

Urologists criticized Johansson's study, alleging that the patients studied were older and had smaller tumors than the patients on whom they operate. Urologists claimed that, in the age of the PSA test, they were operating on prostate cancer earlier and therefore must be prolonging life. No one has proven this, however, and history tells us to doubt surgeons.

When routine chest x-rays picked up lung cancer earlier, chest surgeons were willing to operate on the lung cancers found. But surprisingly, controlled studies eventually found that such surgery was doing more harm than good. The surgery had to be abandoned when the truth came out.

A screening test was developed for neuroblastoma, a childhood cancer. Surgeons were willing to operate. Randomized controlled studies later discovered that the surgery was doing more harm than good. The screening test was picking up cancers that didn't need to be operated on.

Randomized Controlled Studies

Because prostate cancer is unique; it's slow-growing and not lethal in the majority of cases, only randomized controlled studies will tell us if the radical prostatectomy works or not.

Radical Prostatectomy Fails the First Randomized Controlled Study

A controlled study of 111 men was done by the Veteran's Administration Cooperative Urological Research Group and reported by Peter Iversen, Paul Madsen, and Donald Corle in 1995.[165] Interestingly, Dr. Donald Gleason, the inventor of the Gleason grading and scoring system for prostate cancer, did the pathological examinations for this study. This study showed no difference in survival between men who underwent the radical prostatectomy and those who underwent watchful waiting even after 23 years of follow-up. The authors said:

> "With a median of 23 years follow-up, this study fails to demonstrate a survival benefit in patients undergoing radical prostatectomy when compared to patients receiving no initial treatment. This was true when looking at each stage separately or combining results from both stages."[166]

That study used an older staging system where those patients with nonpalpable prostate cancer were stage 1 and those with palpable cancer thought to be confined to the

---

[165] Iversen P, Madsen P, and Corle D: Radical Prostatectomy Versus Expectant Treatment for Early Carcinoma of the Prostate. Twenty-three Year Follow-up of a Prospective Randomized Study. *Scandinavian Journal of Urology and Nephrology*. January 1, 1995;Supplement 172:65-72.

[166] Iversen P, Madsen PO, and Corle DK: Radical prostatectomy versus expectant treatment for early carcinoma of the prostate. Twenty-three year follow-up of a prospective randomized trial. *Scandinavian Journal of Urology and Nephrology*. 1995 Supplement, Jan 1;172:65-72. Quoted with signed, written permission.

prostate were stage 2. This study's conclusions are difficult to overemphasize, in the author's words:

> "Based on the data available today, radical prostatectomy cannot be considered as a proven superior treatment for clinically localized PC [prostate cancer], and we find that deferred therapy remains a reasonable treatment option for these patients. If aggressive therapy is contemplated in younger patients with a considerable life expectancy, the choice of treatment must be the patient's based on meticulous information about the complications and adverse effects and the fact that any gain of the treatment, if present at all, will not accrue for maybe 10-15 years or longer."[167]

The authors additionally concluded:

> "The explosive increase in use of the radical prostatectomy must in our minds be regarded with skepticism."[168]

One oncologist, Dr. Robert Leibowitz, summed up the situation:

> "If radical prostatectomies worked, the data would be there. The reason the data is not

---

[167] Iversen P, Madsen PO, and Corle DK: Radical prostatectomy versus expectant treatment for early carcinoma of the prostate. Twenty-three year follow-up of a prospective randomized study. *Scand J Urol Nephrol.* Suppl. 1995 Jan 1; 172: 65-72. Quoted with signed, written permission.

[168] Iversen P, Madsen PO, and Corle DK: Radical prostatectomy versus expectant treatment for early carcinoma of the prostate. Twenty-three year follow-up of a prospective randomized study. *Scand J Urol Nephrol Suppl.* 1995 Jan 1; 172: 65-72. Quoted with signed, written permission.

there is because radical prostatectomies don't work."[169]

Dr. Leibowitz, who has a web site at ProstateWeb.com, refined his position in 2004 by saying:

"No prospective randomized trial has ever found radical prostatectomy to be both necessary and effective."[170]

Radical Prostatectomy Fails a Second Randomized Controlled Study

The radical prostatectomy failed a second randomized controlled study, which was published in 2002 by Holmberg et al.[171] The Holmberg study followed 695 men diagnosed with prostate cancer between 1989 and 1999. The men had stage T1b, T1c, or T2 and were randomly assigned to watchful waiting or the radical prostatectomy.

After an average follow-up period of 6.2 years, the authors concluded ". . . there was no significant difference between surgery and watchful waiting in terms of overall survival."

The conclusion, based on the two controlled studies we have today, is the radical prostatectomy does not extend the lifespan of the prostate cancer patient. And worse, it always harms men with its side effects.

---

[169] Robert Leibowitz, MD, Compassionate Oncology Medical Group, Tarzana, California. 1994. Available at: http://rattler.cameron.edu/prostate/leibowitz/DrLeib2.html.
[170] Leibowitz, Robert. Email to the author. August 10, 2004. Used with permission.
[171] Holmberg L, Bill-Axelson A, Helgesen F, Salo JO, Folmerz P, Haggman M, Andersson SO, Spangberg A, Busch C, Nordling S, Palmgren J, Adami HO, Johansson JE, Norlen BJ; Scandinavian Prostatic Cancer Group Study Number 4. A randomized trial comparing radical prostatectomy with watchful waiting in early prostate cancer. *New England Journal of Medicine*. 2002:Sep 12;347(11):781-789.

The Radical Prostatectomy Fails a Third Randomized Controlled Trial

Urologist W. Reid Pitts

Princeton and Harvard trained urologist W. Reid Pitts, Jr., MD, FACS, wrote an outstanding letter-to-the-editor of the *Journal of Urology* lambasting the radical prostatectomy.[172] When interviewed he said:

> "Although I did the first ever nerve sparing radical prostatectomy at New York-Cornell Hospital, I've abandoned the radical prostatectomy for my prostate cancer patients. There is always a better treatment option. Urologists need to tell the truth and do what's right based on the medical literature. It's a mistake that urologists don't give up their patients unless it's a hopeless situation, when clearly the patients that are being operated on could be better served by other therapies."[173]

Dr. Pitts also wrote a letter to the editor of the Journal of National Cancer Institute that could not be any clearer:

> "Any apparent 'cure' of prostate cancer by surgery will happen despite the surgery and

---

[172] Pitts WR Jr.: Re:Editorial: The Prostate Puzzle. *Journal of Urology.* 1998;159:1270.

[173] Pitts WR Jr.: Telephone conversation with the author 6/15/1999. Quoted with signed, written permission.

be the result of the biology of the cancer and/or lead time bias."[174]

Lead-Time Bias

Lead-time bias! Your urologist probably hasn't told you a lot about it. Lead-time bias gives some doctors a wonderful way to tell lies and damn lies about prostate cancer.

What happens is that if you suddenly diagnose a disease earlier, you can make it look like some treatment is working better when it is not. Suppose "Ralph" had prostate cancer at age 70, had a radical prostatectomy, and died at age 75.

Now suppose that the PSA test is invented and Ralph has his prostate cancer discovered five years earlier at age 65. He undergoes a radical prostatectomy and still dies at age 75.

Nothing has changed for Ralph, he dies at age 75 in either case, but his survival from diagnosis has increased from 5 years to 10 years, statistically it's a fake success; that's lead-time bias. The reality is that Ralph does worse, because he suffers the side effects of surgery for 10 years instead of 5.

Length-Time bias

The prostate cancer literature also suffers from length-time bias. Length-time bias means picking up cancers that are so small and innocuous that they would never harm a man during his lifetime. Such a man doesn't need operated on, yet he is, and he is counted as a cure, when no cure was needed!

---

[174] Pitts WR Jr.: Letter-to-the-Editor: Outcome Research After Radical Retropubic Prostatectomy for Prostate Cancer. *Journal of the National Cancer Institute.* 1998;90:1107. Quoted with signed, written permission.

Steven J. Milloy MHS, JD, LLM, a lawyer and biostatistician, who publishes the "Junk Science Home Page" on the Internet, talks about both lead-time bias and length-time bias. He says:

> "Advances in tumor detection techniques and broader criteria used to define the disease have allowed more prostate tumors to be found. This translates directly into increased incidence and prevalence of prostate cancer. But, paradoxically, these improved detection techniques have confounded the ability to assess the efficacy of treatment. While improved detection techniques and broader criteria have improved the ability to detect *lethal* tumors, they have also improved the ability to detect *nonlethal* tumors. Not only does a *nonlethal* tumor count as a cancer, but it goes in the survival column as well [length-time bias]. Also, improved detection techniques find tumors earlier. Earlier tumor detection means longer survival times in cases of lethal tumors [lead-time bias]. So more cancer is found (good for fearmongers) and more cancer is cured (good for physicians), but nothing has really changed. The public gets bamboozled again!"[175]

Statistics

In my 20 years of research on prostate cancer, I have identified less than a dozen people who truly understand the statistics behind prostate cancer—and most of these people are not urologists. One of the reasons for this is that urologists cannot step outside their "observer bias." They

---

[175] Milloy, Steven: Are Cancer Survival Rates Increasing? *The Junk Science Home Page*. 1996. Available at http://www.junkscience.com/news/cancer-rates.html. Quoted and edited with signed, written permission.

are surgeons who are trained to do surgery and they interpret studies about surgery more favorably than other people do.

I feel that the number one problem with the specialty of urology is its emphasis on surgery. Unlike other areas of medicine that are clearly divided into medical and surgical halves, such as neurology and neurosurgery, or cardiology and cardiac surgery, the prostate is "owned" by urologists, and urologists are surgeons first and foremost. As a result, there has been a dangerous emphasis on surgery when it comes to treating prostate cancer, without the necessary controlled studies being done to ensure safety and efficacy. Bias in favor of surgery based on inadequate studies permeates the urological literature.

The randomized controlled study is the standard in medicine, and has been since 1940, but urologists seldom do such studies. If you study one man it's a case report. If you study several men it's a case series. This is usually as far as urologists go. They do a case series studies with no control group.

There are striking examples in the urological literature where urologists have done case series studies on the radical prostatectomy, proclaiming they have cured prostate cancer, when in fact, controlled studies show that they have not cured anybody.

Where is the "cure" in such situations? In any event the radical prostatectomy is always a sacrifice, never a cure.

I'll give you an example. One patient wrote up his case history for the *Journal of Urology*. He reported mild urinary incontinence and impotence. He has received collagen injections for his incontinence and has to use penile injections and a vacuum pump to get erections.[176] Should men who have outcomes like this be telling other men that they were "cured" of their prostate cancer?

---

[176] Howe RJ: Prostate Cancer: A patient's perspective. *Journal of Urology.* November 1994;152:1700-1703.

Selection Bias

The prostate cancer literature suffers from selection bias. The healthiest patients with the smallest cancers are usually selected for surgery by urologists. This leaves the sicker patients for the radiation therapists and cryosurgeons. That's unfair in my opinion.

The Money

There's also the money. Urologists charged as much as $8,710 in 1994 for a radical prostatectomy; in fact, the average charge that year was $6,450.[177] The flipside of that coin, as urologist themselves have discussed with me, is that many in the profession don't want anything to do with medical problems such as prostatitis because they only pay an office visit rate—say 50 dollars—that might not even cover their office overhead costs. A Medicare prostatitis visit, one urologist told me, is hardly worth seeing, while you can get rich doing Medicare radical prostatectomies.

Prostate Cancer-Specific Survival

Another way the statistics are misleading is the use of prostate cancer-specific survival. It's wrong not to report "overall survival" in prostate cancer studies. You can have a 100 percent prostate cancer-specific survival in a study, and meanwhile the overall survival is zero! Prostate cancer-specific survival makes surgery look better.

Say you take 100 men who have prostate cancers that are so small they will never need surgery, but being a urologist, you do a radical prostatectomy on all of them. They all eventually die of something other than prostate cancer. You have 100 percent prostate-cancer specific survival, because nobody died of prostate cancer!

---

[177] Mushinski M: Average Charges for a Radical Prostatectomy and a Transurethral Resection of the Prostate (TURP): Geographic Variations. *Oncology*. August 1996;10(8):1162-1179.

Suppose you controlled this same study with an identical group of 100 men who also all had small, irrelevant, prostate cancers. The men in this arm of the study would only be watched until they all also died of something other than their prostate cancer.

When you compare the surgery group with the control group, you find that the increase in overall survival from surgery is zero! The prostate cancer-specific way of reporting survival makes surgery look 100-percent successful, while the correct way to report survival shows that surgery is worthless!

Publishing only prostate cancer-specific survival focuses on what is important to urologists instead of what is important to men with prostate cancer. At a minimum, the data should be reported both ways, showing both overall survival and prostate cancer-specific survival. After all, it's overall survival that's important to men. Here's what an expert says about the situation in the *Journal of the American Medical Association*:

> "Cause-specific survival is an imaginary number that is open to ascertainment bias and only distantly related to quantities a patient might consider centrally important . . . ."[178]

The Radical Prostatectomy is Like the Frontal Lobotomy

The frontal lobotomy, brain surgery for mental illness, was introduced in 1936. It became a fad in the United States in the 1940s and 1950s and came to be called the radical frontal lobotomy.[179] It raised ethical concerns,[180]

---

[178] Fryback DG, Albertsen PC, and Storer BE: Letter-to-the Editor, Prostatectomy and Survival Among Men with Clinically Localized Prostate Cancer. JAMA 1996;276:1723-1724. Available at http://www.ama-assn.org/sci-pubs/journals/archive/jama/vol_276/no_21/letter_5.htm. Quoted with signed, written permission.

[179] Ballantine HT Jr: Historical Overview of psychosurgery and its problematic. *Acta Neurochir.* Suppl (Wien) 1988;44:125-128.

however, because it destroyed patients' brains. Nonetheless, surgeons promoted this "psychosurgery" and "technical improvements" in the technique of doing the radical frontal lobotomy proliferated.[181] Just like today with the radical prostatectomy, some surgeons became celebrities for improving the frontal lobotomy.

The press played a major role in promoting the lobotomy, readily publishing the results of uncontrolled studies furnished by the "experts," just as the press does today with respect to the radical prostatectomy.[182] Eventually, controlled studies demonstrated that the frontal lobotomy doesn't work and that it was doing people more harm than good. The parallels between the radical frontal lobotomy and the radical prostatectomy are so striking it's hard to imagine why doctors and patients have not learned more from history. As they say, if you don't know history, you are doomed to repeat it.

The Failure Rate

The outright failure rate for the radical prostatectomy is high. You can see failure rates as high as 50 percent in some studies. For example, a study out of Northwestern University in Chicago looked at the records of 394 men who achieved undetectable PSA levels after their radical prostatectomies. All the men underwent surgery between 1980 and 1991. Of the 394 men, 133 (34 percent) had recurrence of prostate cancer.[183]

---

[180] Diering SL and Bell WO: Functional neurosurgery for psychiatric disorders: a historical perspective. *Stereotact Funct Neurosurg* 1991;57(4):175-194.

[181] Swayze VW 2nd: Frontal Leukotomy and related psychosurgical procedures in the era before antipsychotics (1935-1954): a historical overview. *Am J Psychiatry*. April 1995;152(4):505-515.

[182] Dorman J: The history of psychosurgery. *Texas Medicine*. July 1995;91(7):54-61.

[183] Oefelein MG, Smith N, Carter M, Dalton D, Schaeffer A: The incidence of prostate cancer progression with undetectable serum prostate specific antigen in a series of 394 radical prostatectomies. *Journal of Urology*. 1995;154(6):2128-2131.

In a Mayo Clinic study in which 261 men had wide radical prostatectomies, the pathology reports after surgery showed that the prostate cancers were confined to the prostate in every case. However, cancer recurred in 20 percent of men within 9.4 years.[184]

Dr. Patrick Walsh, the inventor of the anatomic approach to the radical prostatectomy operated on 820 men from April 8, 1982 to January 1, 1990.[185] How many men failed his operation? This turns out to be a difficult number to determine, because it's not clearly stated in his paper.

The simple answer is that 167 of 721 men failed Dr. Walsh's radical prostatectomy. That's 23 percent! More disturbing is that the failure rate could be higher than that because Dr. Walsh operated on 820 men. Where did 99 of them go? It seems clear from the paper that 20 more failures were dropped from the study. That means that 187 of 742 men failed Dr. Walsh's radical prostatectomy; that's 25 percent. We still have 78 men who have disappeared from the statistics. If they are all failures that means that 78 + 20 + 167 of 820 men failed Dr. Walsh's radical prostatectomy. That is a 32 percent failure rate. My conclusion is that for the first 820 men he operated on, Dr. Walsh had a failure rate between 23 to 32 percent.

The Celebrity Athlete

According to newspaper reports, a famous athlete had two elevated PSA tests and two negative biopsies for prostate cancer, before a third biopsy showed that he had prostate cancer. The celebrity athlete underwent a radical prostatectomy. Press reports appeared naming the doctor,

---

[184] Montgomery BT, Nativ O, Blute ML, Farrow GM, Myers RP, Zincke H, Therneau TM, Lieber MM: Stage B prostate adenocarcinoma. Flow cytometric nuclear DNA ploidy analysis. *Archives of Surgery.* 1990 Mar;125(3):327-331.
[185] Epstein JI, Partin AW, Sauvageot J, and Walsh PC: Prediction of Progression Following Radical Prostatectomy: A Multivariate Analysis of 721 Men with Long-term Follow-up. *American Journal of Surgical Pathology.* 1996;20(3):286-292.

and the hospital, as if they had received a celebrity endorsement.

Later, news reports indicated that the celebrity athlete underwent radiation therapy treatments, because his PSA level rose after surgery. This usually means that prostate cancer was not completely removed by surgery. After a radical prostatectomy, the PSA should go to zero and stay at zero, unless the cancer returns.

I'm not naming names, but men who receive surgery and then radiation are mutilated by two procedures. I see this more and more as surgery fails. We have to ask, wouldn't radiation therapy in the first place have been better?

Unnecessary Radical Prostatectomies

There are various circumstances in which radical prostatectomies are performed unnecessarily. One is largely unavoidable and occurs when, despite a full work-up indicating that the cancer is confined to the prostate, it turns out at surgery that the disease has already escaped the prostate. The odds of this are much higher than one might think. In a Medicare study where 3,173 men underwent radical prostatectomy over 40 percent of men did not have organ-confined prostate cancer.[186]

Urologist Thomas Stamey has written that as many as 50 percent of RPs are unnecessary, either because the prostate cancer is too small and not aggressive enough to have needed surgery, or because it is so aggressive that it has already broken out of the prostate.[187]

---

[186] Grace L. Lu-Yao, Arnold L. Potosky, Peter C. Albertsen, John G. Wasson, Michael J. Barry, John E. Wennberg: Follow-up Prostate Cancer Treatments after Radical Prostatectomy: A Population-Based Study. *Journal of the National Cancer Institute.* 1996;88(3/4):166-73.

[187] Stamey, TA: Prostate Cancer: Who Should be Treated? Oncolink Web site 1995. Available at:
http://cancer.med.upenn.edu/disease/prostate/treatment/stamey.html.

A 2004 study looked at 1095 men with localized prostate cancer who underwent radical prostatectomy. During the 5-year study period, 27 men (2.2 percent) died of prostate cancer, and prostate cancer reoccurred in 366 of the men (33.4 percent). Summing those up, the radical prostatectomy failed in 35.6 percent of the men. It could also be argued that the 57 men (5.2%) who died of other causes during the study period also didn't benefit from their radical prostatectomy.[188]

A reprehensible situation involves performing the RP upon men whose cancer has already spread, as indicated by pre-operative testing, or according to pre-operative predictive tables that give sky-high odds that the cancer is already out of the prostate. Too often this information is ignored, or men are never told about it. There have been situations in which men have had a 90 percent chance that their cancers had spread outside the prostate, but were still given radical prostatectomies. Unless informed, men are clueless about these situations.

The Internet abounds with the case histories posted by men whose RPs have failed. Often the pre-operative data for these men showed that the operation probably should not have been done in the first place. Examples can be found in the medical literature also. One British urologist, Gordon Williams, actually complains in the *British Journal of Urology* about his colleagues operating on men over 75 years of age, and on patients with positive lymph nodes.[189]

One man I know of is particularly furious because his surgery was unnecessary. What made him irate was discovering, after the fact, that his pre-operative CT scan report had shown his cancer to be out of the prostate, but his urologist had operated on him anyway. He calls it the worst joke of his life. He woke up with a "garden hose"

[188] D'Amico AV, Chen MH, Roehl KA, Catalona WJ. Preoperative PSA velocity and the risk of death from prostate cancer after radical prostatectomy. *New England Journal of Medicine*. 2004 Jul 8;351(2):125-35.
[189] Williams G, MS FRCS, Consultant Urologist Hammersmith Hospitals, Commentary, *British Journal of Urology*. 1996;78:911-920, p. 920.

(urinary catheter) coming out of his penis that was sutured to his foreskin. His urologist had done a nerve-sparing operation that was of no use because the cancer was already systemic and the poor man was immediately placed on hormone blockade, which destroyed his libido. Sex for him is impossible. He is so incontinent that any attempts to make love results in him and his wife both wet with urine.

> "I am a 51-year-old white male with a loving supportive spouse and family. I [have] suffered the agonies of incontinence, impotence, anger, rage etc. for the past three and 1/2 years. I too, regret the day I had surgery [a radical prostatectomy]. If I had to do it all over again I would say, 'NO.' My quality of life is so different. . ."[190]

Unfortunately the harms of the radical prostatectomy are far better known and clear cut than the benefits, which in fact, have not yet been shown to exist in a controlled study.

The British National Health Service cited impotence, incontinence, postoperative death, and psychological disturbances from having radical prostatectomies as outweighing any possible benefit.

Urologist W. Scott McDougal writes:

> "Most physicians just can't explain what it's like to recover from a prostatectomy, convey the personal embarrassment of total incontinence, or relate the psychological impact of impotence quite as graphically as those who have lived through them."[191]

---

[190] Name withheld. Quoted with permission.
[191] W. Scott McDougal, MD with P.J. Skerrett. *Prostate Disease*. Copyright 1996 by The General Hospital Corporation. Page 120. The book is part of a series by the Massachusetts General Hospital and is published by Times Books. Dr. McDougal is Chief of Urology at MGH and Professor of Surgery at Harvard Medical School. Quoted with signed, written permission.

Indeed, to critics of the operation, the RP reduces quality of life so immediately and so significantly that the operation had better increase lifespan significantly or else they see no possible net gain in years of "life worth living."

I consider the radical prostatectomy, based on the studies we have today, to be one of the biggest medical scams of all time.

The Wrong Reasons for Surgery

When you find out you have prostate cancer, a dark cloud of doom may descend upon you. You may say or think, "I just can't live with cancer inside me!" If you just can't bear the thought of living with cancer inside you, think again, because of the slow-growing nature of most prostate cancer, many men live with prostate cancer inside them just fine; it's only in a minority of men that prostate cancer is lethal.

Only 7.5 percent of men in the USA who have prostate cancer die from it. Unfortunately the psychology of prostate cancer is such that, despite the statistics, most men seem certain that they are going to die from prostate cancer.

Fortify your bunker! When it comes to prostate cancer not only do you face misinterpretation of medical statistics, you face psychological warfare on many fronts.

Because You Can't Stand Cancer Inside of You

Over and over again, at support groups and on the Internet, I have heard men say that they chose surgery because they cannot stand the thought of having cancer inside of them. I wish I could express how irrational this is. Such men need to understand that it is far better to have a slow-growing innocuous cancer inside them than to destroy their quality of life trying to get it out.

Your Wife, Kids, and Dog

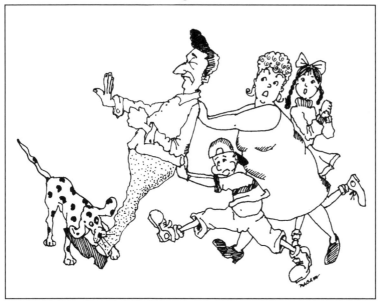

Figure 22. I often see men pushed into the wrong choice by their wife and kids. (Artist: Jun Macam)

I've heard wives say, "Honey, you've got to have surgery," and children say "Dad, you've gotta have surgery." It's striking how often it's the family that can't stand the thought of dad living with prostate cancer inside him—as if he were contagious!

Yet statistically, it's completely rational to consider leaving prostate cancer untreated if the odds are that it's the slow-growing kind, or to treat it by some less harmful method than surgery.

Many men who want to choose watchful waiting, hormone blockade, seeds, radiation, or cryoablation, instead of surgery, often find that their family is less than supportive—even aghast. There's a serious lack of education going on here. It's a crime when people who know virtually nothing about prostate cancer statistics psychologically pressure another person into what may be a horrible decision. Remember that surgery drastically alters a man's quality of life, and that surgery has failed to extend life in two randomized controlled studies.

Strangers

Strangers often aren't helpful either. A line some men who chose watchful waiting sometimes hear when sharing their story of prostate cancer is "How can you stand that cancer inside you?" Outsiders just don't get it. It's better to leave slow-growing cancer inside you than to undergo harmful, unnecessary surgery. The problem is knowing with certainty, whether or not, you have slow-growing prostate cancer.

Because of the Surgeon's Salvage Argument

Urologists tell too many men, rather self-servingly, that if their RP fails they can always have radiation therapy later. This is the "salvage argument" that is sometimes used on patients. It makes little sense that the fact that the RP often fails is made into a reason for having one!

Surgeons make men feel like they are giving up an option if they chose radiation therapy over surgery. It's true that if men have radiation therapy a subsequent RP is a poor idea because the radiation may cause too much tissue damage for good healing to take place after surgery. On the other hand, when the RP fails many men are now getting radiation for the failed operation. Why not just undergo radiation in the first place? Wouldn't that route be better for many men rather than having the side effects of two treatments?

The most important thing is to choose the therapy that has the best chance of curing prostate cancer and to do that therapy first, so that men don't end up with the side effects of two major treatments. Avoid having a radical prostatectomy that fails and then having to have another treatment on top of it. Don't plan for failure. Pick the best therapy for your cancer up front!

Because of Prostate Cancer Death

I am well aware of the psychological games used to encourage men to have surgery. Some urologists have told men that, "You don't want to die from prostate cancer; it's a terrible way to go."

Such statements are hardly an argument for having the RP when the operation has failed to extend life in two controlled studies. Yet, when coming from the mouths of urologists, such statements often have the effect of promoting surgery. I am not aware of any controlled study that proves that patients die a better death after undergoing a radical prostatectomy, but I am aware of many studies that prove that men who have an RP lead a worse life!

If you think you have to have surgery because dying from prostate cancer is terrible, ask yourself what the operation will do to your quality of life and if it will extend your life. Ask yourself if urologists bear a portion of the responsibility for the "terribleness" of prostate cancer death because of inappropriate pain management. Do you see urologists sitting by the bedside to the bitter end, maximizing pain management for men dying from prostate cancer, or do you see them being too busy operating on other patients to properly attend dying men? Do you see urologists offering proper hormone blockade therapy?

The best course of action is to give men the finest possible treatment based on science, not to give them treatment based upon manipulating their fear of death.

I don't want to die and neither do you. We both need to face our worst fears in order to better deal with the alternatives and options for treating prostate cancer. I've seen people die and prostate cancer death has no franchise on undesirability.

One physician, who corresponded with me about how urologists threaten men with a terrible prostate cancer death if they don't undergo surgery immediately, called such behavior, "A primitive and unethical form of marketing."

Because of a High Gleason Score

"You have a high Gleason score, you'd better have surgery." We wish that the Gleason score would help us more than it does. The fact is that when men have a high Gleason score, surgery may be too late, and with a low Gleason score most men don't need surgery. We have no good way of picking out the few men, who urologists claim exist, that in theory have just the right prostate cancer to operate on. The Gleason score doesn't allow us to perfectly distinguish aggressive from non-aggressive prostate cancer even though it does suggest some tendencies. This is a difficult concept but Dr. Stephen Woolf words the dilemma perfectly:

> "For now, neither PSA values nor histologic findings can predict with certainty whether a newly diagnosed prostate cancer will progress or remain latent."[192]

Some men are told, "If you don't have surgery right away the cancer might spread!" Because most prostate cancer is slow-growing, most men have time to stop and weigh their options. Many men today go on hormone blockade while weighing their options for local treatment of the tumor. If there is one lesson that has been learned with prostate cancer, it is that it may be better to take your time and make the right choice than to make the wrong one.

---

[192] Woolf, Steven H, MD, MPH: Current Concepts: Screening for Prostate Cancer with Prostate-Specific Antigen. *New England Journal of Medicine.* 1995;Vol. 333 No. 21, pp1401-1405. Copyright 1995 Massachusetts Medical Society. All rights Reserved. Quoted with signed, written permission.

Because You're Too Young

"You're too young to have prostate cancer. You'd better get a radical prostatectomy." This argument is somewhat of an appeal to your vanity. Simply because prostate cancer is being picked up in younger men because of the PSA test, does this mean that it's more amenable to surgery? Surgeons like to think so, but in fact operating on prostate cancer in younger men has not been proven to be beneficial in controlled studies.

Besides, one large study shows younger men do better than older men with watchful waiting. The Chodak study, for instance, which looked at pooled data from 828 patients, found that younger men on watchful waiting did better than older men on watchful waiting for low-grade and medium-grade prostate cancer in terms of 10-year survival.[193] Men younger than age 61 with low-grade (Gleason 2, 3, 4) or medium-grade (Gleason 5, 6, 7) prostate cancer had a prostate cancer-specific survival of 97 percent at 10 years while on watchful waiting. By contrast, men aged 61 or older with low-grade (Gleason 2, 3, 4) or medium-grade prostate cancer had a 10-year prostate cancer-specific survival of 84 percent while on watchful waiting.

Any increased survival reported from doing radical prostatectomies on younger men may be completely due to length-time, lead-time, and other biases. Many men with early prostate cancer might never be affected by it during their lifetime. Oncologist Stephen Strum says:

"Recommendations for RP should NEVER be made because of young age but BECAUSE OF LOCAL THERAPY BEING APPROPRIATE FOR THAT PARTICULAR PATIENT. I type in

---

[193] Chodak GW, Thisted RA, Gerber GS, Johansson JE, Adolfsson J, Jones GW, Chisholm GD, Moskovitz B, Livne PM, and Warner J: Results of conservative management of clinically localized prostate cancer. *New England Journal of Medicine*. January 27, 1994;330(4):242-248.

caps because that message must be shouted from the highest medical office tops. You select the patient for appropriate therapy based on clinical and pathologic findings. You may not choose to do a RP if the patient is old and/or infirm but you don't choose a local therapy just because the patient is young."[194]

It boils down to this: If urologists are going to operate on young men with very early prostate cancer, are urologists sure that they are extending their lives? Are urologists sure that they have a cancer that actually needs treatment and don't have an incidental cancer? We know that surgery will damage their quality of life for the rest of their days. And if we operate on a young man with larger, higher-grade prostate cancer, we shouldn't fail to address the possibility that he has systemic disease, even if our tests aren't sensitive enough to discover it.

Debulking

"You should have your tumor debulked." Some surgeons justify performing the radical prostatectomy on patients by telling men that it's a good idea to take away part of the cancer even if they can't get it all. I've heard men say exactly this in prostate cancer support groups. "The surgeon couldn't get it all but I feel better having the bulk of it out."

Removing only part of a man's prostate cancer is simply adding insult to injury. There is the possibility that by removing some of the main tumor, you also remove its hormones, and those hormones may be suppressing metastases from growing. Removal may allow the metastases to start growing.

---

[194] Strum, Stephen. Re: [p2p] Perineural Invasion, RPP versus RRP? *The Patient to Physician Mailing List.* June 23, 1997. Quoted with signed, written permission.

To paraphrase Urologist William Lynes the problem with debulking prostate cancer is that those caner cells left behind still have the potential to cause death.[195]

Worse, if you only get part of the cancer out with surgery, the man is doomed to other therapies and side effects on top of the surgery that failed.

Long-Term Data

I have heard some people argue that, "Only the radical prostatectomy has long-term data available." The first five hundred men to undergo the modern version of the radical prostatectomy were operated on at Johns Hopkins between 1982 and 1988. This means that the data on the modern version of the RP is pretty recent.

Large-scale use of the PSA test only began around 1985, and most other therapies for prostate cancer gained steam around that time as well. It's purely a myth that there exists a vast amount of long-term data demonstrating that the RP is superior to other therapies. Sure the RP has long-term data; data that shows it doesn't work!

The fact that the RP has a longer track record than some other therapies is not helpful at all in my opinion since no controlled study has proven that the RP works, only that it doesn't.

Sex or Death

Gravely disturbing is the "what do you want, sex or death?" approach of encouraging men to have a radical prostatectomy. Men are sometimes wrongly made to believe that they must either undergo a radical prostatectomy and give up sex or die. It's really a choice between an unknown and possibly nonexistent benefit from the radical

---

[195] Lynes, William, MD: Radiotherapy is not Indicated. Re:[p2p] Going off LHRH with Radiation. 97-07-20 21:40:35 EDT. Available at: http://users.alphainfo.com/wlynes.

prostatectomy versus sexual dysfunction for the rest of your life.

Sadly, the trend is to do the radical prostatectomy on younger men, who are all the more likely to feel that the RP has affected their sex lives.

Based on what I know today, I would not have a radical prostatectomy in my 30s, 40s, 50s, 60s, 70s, 80s, or 90s.

The Stockholm Syndrome

It's hard to explain why men accept the side effects of the radical prostatectomy when no controlled study has shown it to extend life. After being told they have cancer, men opt for surgery with inadequate knowledge about what surgery really entails. Afterwards, when better informed, many men refuse to face the possibility that their surgery was unnecessary. Instead, they loudly defend the operation, despite their diminished sexual function and other distressing side effects.

In defense of their operation, urologists have been giving men "satisfaction surveys." According to such surveys, the majority of men who have the radical prostatectomy would have it again. The flaw with such studies is that those men believe the radical prostatectomy cured them of their prostate cancer. If such surveys were done in the context that the radical prostatectomy does not extend life, satisfaction levels would be much different!

Consider the magnified humiliation of radical prostatectomy patients. Not only has their money been taken, but their penises have been crippled and their sex lives have been largely destroyed. Few men are going to be able to stand up in public and admit to not understanding the statistics before surgery. Quite the opposite; the situation is so painful they feel they must claim that the *New England Journal of Medicine*, the *Journal of the American Medical Association* (JAMA), the Centers for

Disease Control, and the entire British Health Service, just for starters, are all wrong.

Recovery, such as it is, from the radical prostatectomy normally takes one to two years. Some men will regain control of their urinary continence, but none will completely recover normal sexual function. All post-RP patients are sterile; they don't ejaculate any semen. All will have smaller penises. Many won't be able to achieve as many erections, and those who do will have partial erections only. There is no question that the radical prostatectomy demands a heavy price.

Michael Korda in his book, *Man to Man: Surviving Prostate Cancer*, describes meeting Seymour, the CEO of a company who had his surgery at the hands of a urologist considered to be eminent. Korda describes Seymour as "worshipping his surgeon."[196] As Korda questions Seymour the truth slowly emerges. About incontinence Seymour says, "I'm fine now, except when I laugh hard, then I wet my pants a bit, but what the hell, who knows, who cares?" About sex, Seymour says, "Of course you don't get a *full* erection at this stage. My New York urologist, the guy who took out the catheter, he told me, 'It won't be like it was when you were seventeen, *bubbe*, but with any luck you'll have a *stuffable* erection, if you know what I mean.'" Korda then notes that Seymour laughed at his own joke but not too hard.[197]

A Conversation About the RP

What men don't know about prostate cancer is much more than a trifling problem. Imagine this conversation between a prostate cancer patient (loosely based on some real conversations) and me:

---

[196] Korda, Michael. *Man to Man: Surviving Prostate Cancer*. New York: Random House, 1996. p. 58 - 63. Quoted with signed, written permission.
[197] Korda, Michael. *Man to Man: Surviving Prostate Cancer*. New York: Random House, 1996. p. 58 - 63. Quoted with signed, written permission.

"Hi, I'm Doctor Hennenfent."

"Hi, I'm a sixty-one year old male who had an RP. I'm incontinent, impotent, and I'm on hormone blockade, but I'm glad I had the RP. The side effects everybody talks about are no big deal. I can live with them."

"Are you sure you made the right decision?"

"Yes. I'm capable of making an important decision like whether or not to have a radical prostatectomy, and I made mine," he says.

"I think," I say, "men would be able to make a good decision about prostate cancer if they had the right information, but most men are given incorrect information. I think it would take most men several years of studying to make a good decision about prostate cancer treatment . . ."

He rolls his eyes so I stop talking.

"So," he says.

"Well, most men don't ever really understand the situation."

"So," he says again.

The rest of the conversation, I don't say out loud, but I imagine how it might go.

"You're incontinent and impotent," I want to say, but don't. "How can you think that you are an advertisement for a radical prostatectomy? And, you are on hormone blockade, which means that your radical prostatectomy failed. You definitely had needless surgery and you could have known it, if you had been informed."

"I have a kind and considerate urologist," he would probably say, aghast, which is exactly what many men do tell me, no matter how badly their urologist mutilated them.

"Did your urologist tell you that in the longest controlled study ever done on the issue, after 23 years of follow-up, the radical prostatectomy failed to show any benefit for men? Did he tell you that the second randomized controlled study also showed no increase in survival? Did he tell you about doctors publishing in almost every major medical journal speculation that the RP may not work, or does more harm than good?"

I don't engage in these kinds of conversations if I can avoid them, because I don't want to hurt anyone's feelings. A radical prostatectomy can't be undone. The men that are post radical prostatectomy, that geared up for their major surgery, and are gung ho—you can't tell them that they might have done the wrong thing, not after what it has cost them financially, emotionally, and physically. This book is meant for men before they get a radical prostatectomy. Men are still free to choose the radical prostatectomy, but at least they will be better informed.

We need to look at the RP's failure to extend life, tabulate its side effects, then show men this information and ask, "Are these disabling side effects okay for an operation that hasn't even extended survival in a controlled study?" By presenting the information honestly, I would expect nearly all men and women to say that the radical prostatectomy is an unacceptable treatment for prostate cancer.

Impotent or Incontinent Evangelists

I am frequently amazed about how often it is the impotent man who screams the loudest in favor of the radical prostatectomy. I think this is partly the Stockholm syndrome and partly the inability to accept that a terrible sacrifice did not result in extended survival. One doctor colleague calls the situation "cognitive dissonance."

When men who have underwent a radical prostatectomy eulogize about how great it is, they should first tell exactly what their sexual function is, what their urinary function is, and then list their other side effects, before they begin telling other men why they love having had surgery. Such men should begin with something like, "I am completely impotent, I wear one pad, and the radical prostatectomy has failed to extend life in two controlled studies, but I still believe in it because . . . ." What the post-RP man should never do is extol its virtues while hiding its side effects from other men trying to make a decision. One prostate cancer support group leader wrote me about the problem, saying that such men were like "Lenin's useful idiots" for promoting surgery. That's harsh, but so are the side effects of a radical operation that doesn't extend life.

Urologists Want to Believe that the Radical Prostatectomy Works

Even in face of criticism from academic physicians from other specialties who say the operation remains unproved or doesn't work, urologists want to believe that the radical prostatectomy cures prostate cancer. Urologists want to believe that they can remove the prostate before the cancer spreads. They also want to be believe that the men whose prostates they remove would suffer from their prostate cancer in the future before dying of some other illness. And, let's face it; they probably wouldn't be crazy about their most lucrative operation disappearing.

But if the RP worked without question, every doctor all over the world would always be recommending it, and studies would unequivocally show that men benefit from it. Sadly, this is not the case.

In a now famous quote, urologist Willet Whitmore described the situation perfectly, "Is cure possible for men in whom it is necessary? And is cure necessary for men in whom it is possible?"

Urologists continue to publish uncontrolled studies to support their operation. Don't make your decision on studies that urologists publish. After reviewing a study done in Great Britain touting the radical prostatectomy, another urologist, Dr. Gordon Williams, an editor of the *British Journal of Urology*, wrote:

> "These authors have provided nothing new and particularly no evidence that radical prostatectomy alters the natural history of prostate cancer. They have made unwarranted conclusions from data presented. Surgeons and physicians of influence should use this influence responsibly. Contradictions in their positions and their inability to recognize adequately the lack of proven efficacy is in marked contrast to their willingness to undertake this procedure and must raise questions about their motives."[198]

The data suggests that when a urologist operates on prostate cancer and the operation appears successful, the man operated on had slow-growing prostate cancer and didn't need the operation. When a man has aggressive prostate cancer that needs curing, the surgery has failed before the urologist ever starts cutting, because his cancer has already escaped the prostate.

Urologists

When it comes to prostate cancer and deciding whether to have surgery or not, it's best not to put yourself solely in your urologist's hands. The same man, who will go to 10 car dealerships before buying a car, often fails to

---

[198] Williams G., MS FRCS, Consultant Urologist, Hammersmith Hospitals, NHS Trust, Du Cane Road, London, W12 OHS, UK. Commentary. *British Journal of Urology*. 1996;78:911-920, p. 920. Used with signed, written permission.

realize that urologists can be as self-serving as any car salesman with their advice.

Researchers around the world are critical of urologists in the United States. Many experts see the large number of radical prostatectomies being done in the United States as being driven by profit and not by scientific proof that the operation works. Dr. David Dearnaley of the Royal Mardsen Hospital in London commented in documentary called Cancer Wars that:

> "In North America, it's . . . to be cynical, obviously in the interests of the urological surgeons to perform lots of operations because that's how they earn their money."[199]

It defies the human experience to suggest that the medical profession might be doing something harmful. But we only have to look back in history at unnecessary hysterectomies, tonsillectomies, lung cancer operations, and the frontal lobotomy to know that surgeons make mistakes.

Obviously, surgeons often interpret medical data in a biased fashion. Prostate cancer is a disease that requires you to do your homework. Investigate every avenue. Speak to an oncologist, a radiation seed implant expert, a combined precision irradiation expert, an external beam radiation therapy expert, a hormone blockade expert, and a cryoablation expert, before you decide how, and if you want to be treated. Read and study! You stand to lose your sexual function, your urinary function, and the ability to enjoy the remaining years of your life.

---

[199] Dearnaley, David: Cancer Wars: Part Four. WETA Television, Corporation for Public Broadcasting. Directed and produced by Jenny Barraclough. Written by George Carey. June 1998.

The FDA is Not Protecting You From the RP

Many people assume that the government is protecting them from harmful surgery in the same way that it protects them from harmful drugs. Not so! The FDA does not have regulatory authority over the radical prostatectomy.

Every new drug must undergo a series of successful studies, including randomized controlled trials. Imagine if the radical prostatectomy had to be approved by the FDA before being unleashed upon American men. Would they approve the operation? A letter to the FDA would be a joke:

Dear Food and Drug Administration (FDA):

We have a treatment called the radical prostatectomy, which we would like to submit for FDA approval as a treatment for prostate cancer.

The radical prostatectomy has been studied for about 100 years and is done more than ever today. It's wildly popular among urologists. The RP has undergone two randomized controlled studies, which have shown no increase in overall survival over watchful waiting or placebo.

We know that in 100-years time we should have done more randomized controlled studies, but what can we do? You know how it goes. We're busy.

We *feel* that radical surgery will be shown to work any day now. We've been saying this for years but please bear with us.

Sure, the radical prostatectomy is major surgery and causes sexual dysfunction in 100 percent of the men who undergo it. Sure, it may leave up to 60 percent of men with some degree of urinary incontinence, and of course it causes urinary strictures in about 15 percent of men, but these and all the other side effects are acceptable to us surgeons.

In summary, we, the Urologists of America, would like FDA approval for the radical prostatectomy, which has failed to extend life in randomized controlled studies, but definitely has very harmful side effects. Thank you!

Signed: America's Urologists

Banning the RP

There is a case for banning the radical prostatectomy until it is proven to benefit men in a randomized controlled trial. The cold reality is that many of the world's best medical journals and doctors agree that there is no clear scientific proof that it extends life. Meanwhile the costs in terms of side effects are staggering, not to mention wasted health-care dollars.

Urologists Believe

The radical prostatectomy is essentially never used in some countries, yet some urologists seem determined to make their most lucrative operation work. They are willing to operate on most men with prostate cancer in order to get to the not-yet-proven-to-exist man that might benefit from a radical prostatectomy. Most men are not informed beforehand in a way that conveys the situation adequately. How many men realize that the RP does not extend life according to controlled studies? How many realize that if it does work for a small subset of men, they may have to live 10 or 15 years with sexual dysfunction, decreased libido, a likelihood of incontinence, and other side effects, before seeing their benefit, which may only last a year, or a few years? Oncologist Robert Leibowitz says it well:

"The vast majority of men being diagnosed now by the PSA almost certainly have biologically indolent disease; yet they are being "guided" by well intentioned urologists into having aggressive, unnecessary radical procedures that leave them incontinent and impotent. I do not claim that I have the final and correct answer for the treatment of prostate cancer. But I do know that we have been treating this disease wrong . . . and the side effects are far, far worse than most will acknowledge."[200]

The Press Misinforms Us

Men must remain ever diligent about bad information. Don't get your information from the popular press. It's clear that most health reporters don't understand medical statistics; even worse, they consult urologists. Urologists give statistics that tend to promote their operations.

I see the press repeatedly reporting that surgery cures prostate cancer based on uncontrolled studies. If the press only knew statistics, they would know that they are being fed lies, damn lies, and "bad prostate cancer statistics."

---

[200] Leibowitz, Bob MD: Emerging Concepts Prostate Cancer 1997-2000. Available at http://rattler.cameron.edu/leibowitz/DrLeib8.html. Quoted with signed, written permission.

Six Ways the Radical Prostatectomy May Spread Prostate Cancer

There are theoretical concerns as to why undergoing a radical prostatectomy may actually spread prostate cancer.

1) The Biopsy

One of the proposed theories for how prostate cancer arises is that cells behind partially obstructed prostatic acini evolve into pre-cancerous cells. These pre-cancer cells are called PIN (prostatic intraepithelial neoplasia) cells. Dr. H. Hale Harvey suggests that the process of doing a biopsy can disperse PIN cells into the stroma of the prostate—the tissue between the acini—where they set off prostate cancer. This may explain why repeated biopsies of men who have high-grade PIN cells often finds prostate cancer; the biopsy is actually causing it.[201]

2) Tracking Down the Needle Path

After a biopsy is done, prostate cancer can escape the prostate by following the path left by the needle. One study looked at 350 men who had prostate biopsies and demonstrated prostate cancer trying to escape down the needle path in seven of them and there were also 13 more possible cases of such "tumor tracking" in the study. The

---

[201] H. Hale Harvey MD, PhD, MPH: A Unifying Hypothesis that Links Benign Prostatic Hyperplasia and Prostatic Intraepithelial Neoplasia with Prostate Cancer: Invited Comments. *Pathology Research and Practice*. 1995;191:924-934.

distance the tumors tracked in these patients ranged from 1 mm to 12 mm. It only took an average of 3.5 months for the tumors to track this far. The authors warn that "tumor tracking" along the path left by the biopsy needle is a real phenomenon, which occurs even with the newer thinner biopsy needles.[202]

Most prostate cancers are on the back of the prostate and are already close to the capsule. Do you really want to lay down a path for it to escape beyond the capsule? If a man is almost certain to chose watchful waiting is a biopsy really necessary?

I came across a man who was shown his prostate cancer slides after his radical prostatectomy. He was told, "See, your cancer was trying to escape."

My opinion, based on the information given, was that his cancer was tracking down the needle track left by his biopsy, and might have stayed put if his urologist had not stuck a needle into it.

3) Biopsy Spreads Cells into the Bloodstream

Doing a prostate biopsy spreads prostate cells into the bloodstream. One study found that in 10 percent of men, prostate cells were being released into the bloodstream during the biopsy procedure. This may be a mechanism for spreading prostate cancer throughout the body.[203]

4) Spilling Cancer in the Bed of the Operation

"Don't touch the cancer!"

---

[202] Batasky SS, Walsh PC, and Epstein JI: Needle biopsy associated tumor tracking of adenocarcinoma of the prostate. *Journal of Urology*. May 1991;145:1003-1007.
[203] Moreno, JG, O'Hara SM, Long JP, Veltri RW, Ning X, Alexander AA, Gomella LG: Transrectal ultrasound-guided biopsy causes hematogenous dissemination of prostate cells as determined by RT-PCR. UROLOGY. 1997; 49; 515-520.

Surgeons often use a "no touch" technique during cancer surgery. This is because manipulating some cancers probably spreads them.

Some fascinating studies using highly sensitive DNA techniques suggest that prostate cancer is one of the cancers that should not be touched during surgery. One study found that in about 14 percent of men spillage of malignant cells into the prostate bed probably occurs during surgery.[204]

Another study found that in over 90 percent of cases, prostate cells were being left behind in the bed of the operation site after surgery.[205] This tumor spillage may explain why prostate cancer often returns after surgery.

5) Surgery Spreads Cells into the Bloodstream

Studies have also shown that prostate cells are released into the blood stream during the radical prostatectomy. In one study, prostate cells were shed into the bloodstreams of 25 percent of the men who underwent radical prostatectomies.[206] This may explain distant metastases occurring after a radical prostatectomy.

6) When it Fails the RP Causes a More Aggressive Cancer

There is evidence that if you have a radical prostatectomy, and it fails, the tumor that comes back will be more aggressive than the tumor you started with. A 1997

---

[204] Kassabian VS, Bottles K, Weaver R, Williams RD, Paulson DF, and Scardino PT: Possible mechanism for seeding of tumor during radical prostatectomy. *Journal of Urology.* October 1993;150:1169-1171.

[205] Oeflein MG, Kaul K, Herz B, Blum MD, Holland JM, Keeler TC, Cook WA, Ignatoff JM: Molecular detection of prostate epithelial cells from the surgical field and peripheral circulation during radical prostatectomy. *Journal of Urology.* 1996;155(1):238-242.

[206] Oefelein MG, Kaul K, Herz B, Blum MD, Holland JM, Keeler TC, Cook WA, and Ignatoff JM: Molecular Detection of Prostate Epithelial Cells from the Surgical Field and Peripheral Circulation During Radical Prostatectomy. *Journal of Urology.* January 1996;155:238-242.

article asserts that the growth rates of recurrent cancers after RP are higher than the growth rates of the original parent tumors.[207]

Returning prostate cancer might be more aggressive, because when the parent tumor in the prostate is removed, so is an important hormone. Some doctors believe that the main cancer tumor in the prostate secretes a hormone that keeps the metastatic cells elsewhere in the body from growing rapidly. When the parent tumor is removed, so is this hormone, which allows the metastatic cells to divide unchecked and become more aggressive. If a man has a radical prostatectomy and unknowingly has micrometastases, the removal of the primary tumor may cause the indolent metastases to become uninhibited and grow aggressively.

Weak Evidence that the Radical Prostatectomy Kills

Let's compare a 1994 study of 828 patients who underwent watchful waiting[208] with a 1996 study of 2,758 men who underwent radical prostatectomy.[209] Both of these studies claim to give the best available estimates on survival. Let's also focus on the most common grade of prostate cancer — medium-grade prostate cancer, since most men operated on have that type.

---

[207] Connolly J, et al: Accelerated Tumor Proliferation Rates in Locally Recurrent Prostate Cancer after Radical Prostatectomy. *Journal of Urology*. August 1997;158:515-518.

[208] Chodak GW, Thisted RA, Gerber GS, Johansson JE, Adolfsson J, Jones GW, Chisholm GD, Moskovitz B, Livne PM, and Warner J: "Results of Conservative Management of Clinically Localized Prostate Cancer." *New England Journal of Medicine*. January 24, 1994;330(4)242-248.

[209] Gerber GS, Thisted RA, Scardino PT, Frohmuller HGW, Schroeder GH, Paulson DF, Middleton AW, Rukstalis DB, Smith JA, Schellhammer PF, Ohori M, and Chodak GW: "Results of Radical Prostatectomy in Men with Clinically Localized Prostate Cancer." JAMA. August 28, 1996;276(8):615-619.

	Survival with watchful waiting	Survival after radical prostatectomy
Men with Medium-grade prostate cancer	87%	80%

Men who underwent surgery had 7 percent *less* survival than men who simply underwent watchful waiting—a sign, perhaps, that the radical prostatectomy actually spreads prostate cancer, or causes death by some other means.

Conclusion

We have already documented many ways in which the radical prostatectomy hurts people by way of side effects. We also need to know for sure if the process of getting ready for and undergoing surgery actually spreads cancer, or causes death in some other way.

What I Would Do

I have a higher risk of prostate cancer than most men, because four of my blood-related uncles have had it. What would I do if I were diagnosed with localized prostate cancer?

I want to be crystal clear that when the time comes, I will base my treatment decisions on randomized controlled studies, because when done properly, they provide the truth. Furthermore, my goal will be to maintain the quality of my life, not the length of my life at any cost.

When and if I get localized prostate cancer, I will avoid surgery like the plague. After reviewing the world's literature on the radical prostatectomy, I'm convinced that studies published by urologists are full of lies, damn lies, and biased statistics. The bottom line is that the radical prostatectomy has failed to extend life in two randomized controlled studies involving over 800 men, and with 23 years of follow-up for 111 of those men. Based on the data we have today, the radical prostatectomy for prostate cancer is a sham, oversold, over-advertised, ineffective at extending life, and one of the greatest medical hoaxes of all time.

The randomized controlled study was invented in 1940 and is what separates the medical doctors of western medicine from snake oil salesmen. Instead of doing the proper studies before unleashing their new operation, urologists and institutions that would make money from doing prostate cancer surgery ignored science.

I am convinced that urologists' goals and mine are different. Urologists, as evidenced by the bias in their studies and statements, want to do surgery and perfect surgery. I want to extend my life without sacrificing quality of life. I want to cure prostate cancer while remaining potent and continent. I want a true "cure," not a sacrifice.

Remember my two philosophies: 1) I will allow randomized, controlled trials to dictate my decisions when they are available, and 2) when the proper studies have not been done, I will follow the least harmful path to treatment based on the best studies available.

You must educate yourself and seek as many sources of information as you can, especially those that are not filtered through the prejudiced eyes of the urological profession.

If I get prostate cancer, I will first start watchful waiting. I will quickly follow watchful waiting with active non-invasive therapy (ANIT), part of which means reading the latest and greatest medical studies.

I will almost immediately try PC SPES, if it is available to me, or a similar product. Perhaps, I will consider adding low dose estrogen with a blood thinner to that regimen. I will go with systemic therapies first because it is the metastases of prostate cancer that kill you. I will see how my PSA responds to these therapies, testing my PSA and doing other tests frequently. I will also assess my quality of life, as I continue investigating. I will hope that my systemic therapy will give me time to study the very latest studies, and to interview even more experts.

Next, I will look at local therapies such as cryoablation, radiation seed implants, 3-D conformal radiation, intensity modulated radiation therapy, and every other form of radiation therapy. Because cryoablation and radiation can both be so well focused, if my cancer is particularly small and localized, I will be very tempted to treat locally with one of those therapies. If, the right doctor does my biopsy, and if the prostate cancer is small and accessible, I may chose very limited cryosurgery, or a very focused radiation therapy.

I will always be considering starting hormone blockade regardless of the stage and grade of prostate cancer that I have, and I will be hoping that triple hormone blockade followed by Proscar (finasteride) maintenance, or intermittent hormone blockade, will have been proven to extend life by the time I that I need them. In fact, I will seriously consider bypassing PC SPES and or estrogen and going straight to combined hormone blockade as my first treatment, depending on the results of studies now in progress—especially if such studies show that increased quality-of-life survival can be obtained by being on hormone blockade for a short time, intermittently, or by stopping all the blockade except Proscar maintenance.

I will also seriously consider the strategy of going on double or triple hormone blockade, undergoing a local therapy, and then going off hormone blockade.

I will also pursue prostate cancer vaccines. Vaccines, it is hoped, will soon be used to rev up our body's natural defenses to kill the prostate cancer inside of us.

I will keep my eyes open for promising new therapies such as angiogenesis inhibitors. Angiogenesis inhibitors stop the growth of new blood vessels. These drugs have been used to cure cancer in mice and work is feverishly underway to translate the success in laboratory mice to humans.

I will try to find a place that will work on an individualized vaccine, medication, and herbal plan for me, instead of a program designed for the masses. This means finding a place that will put my cancer in mice, and then will test different agents against those mice that contain my cancer.

With so much happening with hormone blockade, radiation therapies, cryoablation, and potential new therapies, it may be a terrible mistake to let your prostate and seminal vesicles be ripped out during radical surgery. Think of your quality of life as you pursue a cure for prostate cancer. However, you do not have to do what I do. People can look at the same facts and make different decisions, and more importantly, people can look at the same *lack of facts* and make different decisions.

I apologize for my profession. I was taught that doctors must be great scientists and practice medicine based on randomized controlled studies, with proof that therapies work. Do no harm was our dictum. Now, since I have looked over the shoulders of urologists to see what so many of them are doing, I have seen what a joke western medicine can be. Thankfully, I have seen a few heroic urologists—and other specialists—emerge from the unscientific rubble.

Patient Power

This is a book about prostate cancer. It's not supposed to be a book about changing our health-care system. But our health-care system is corrupt, inept, and is killing us.

The PSA Test

Aubrey Pilgrim, in his book *A Revolutionary Approach to Prostate Cancer,* describes going to his doctor for urinary symptoms. He asked his doctor if he should have a PSA test. His doctor didn't seem to think so, because Pilgram's HMO required that a urologist order it. Pilgrim took charge, got his PSA test despite the HMO, and found out that he had prostate cancer.

PSA Test in Canada

Gordon (a pseudonym) wanted to get a PSA test. "The Canadian Health-Care system does not allow it," he was told.

Gordon would eventually go around the Canadian socialized health care system and get a PSA test. It was high. Gordon had prostate cancer, but his diagnosis was delayed by nearly a year by the time he got a private doctor to do the PSA test, another to do a biopsy, and yet another to read his slides.

Cryosurgery

Roger (a composite character) has prostate cancer. He is convinced that cryoablation is the best treatment for him. He sees it as far less dangerous than the major surgery that a radical prostatectomy entails. Also, he thinks it will be more likely to cure his prostate cancer. To his dismay, he finds out that Medicare won't pay for cryoablation.

Roger and others became activists and sued to get Medicare to pay for cryoablation. They felt that urologists were their biggest enemy in getting cryoablation paid for, as they were often the dissenting experts when testimony was given. After an extreme amount of effort by many men to finally get Medicare to pay for cryoablation, it was only a partial victory, because reimbursement was set so low that many doctors couldn't afford to do cryoablation. Many prostate cancer victims blame urologists for sabotaging the reimbursement rate.

Estramustine

Tony (a composite character) is dying from hormone resistant prostate cancer. He believes, as do many physicians in Japan and Europe, that estramustine probably extends life for about six months in men with his type of prostate cancer. Tony would like to have those six months.

But Tony discovers that since estramustine is an oral medication; it's not adequately reimbursed under American insurance schemes, therefore, oncologists in the USA rarely use it. Instead, they stay with injectable drugs, for which they can get reimbursed without a hassle.

Caverject

Blake (a composite character) underwent urological surgery, which left him impotent. The one thing that works for him is Caverject (alprostadil). Blake injects the medication into his penis to get an erection.

The trouble is that only six doses come in a package. To Blake's dismay his Health Maintenance Organization will only pay for one package every 30 days. This means that

Blake is only allowed six erections per month. His HMO literally controls his sex life.

Castration Surgery

A physician writes to his local newspaper, complaining that managed care has mandated that men undergoing castration for prostate cancer must be discharged the same day. Some men need more than one day after undergoing such a cruel operation. Yet, patients and doctors have no power.[210]

Pain Control for a TRUS

Denzel (a composite character) goes to get a transrectal ultrasound in a large New York City hospital. He knows that it will be "uncomfortable," to use the doctor's euphemism for "severely painful," because he has had one before. He wants to have topical lidocaine, the anesthetic applied before the procedure.

"We don't give it," is the answer he receives. The hospital has a policy about how transrectal ultrasounds are done. Having no choice, Denzel undergoes the 30-minute procedure, which was far more painful than it needed to be.

Pain Control for a Biopsy

Hank (a composite character) goes in for a biopsy to check for prostate cancer. He wants intravenous sedation, because he knows it's going to be painful. "You don't need it," the doctor says. Hank insists that he wants it. "Nobody has sedation for a biopsy," he is told.

The truth is that sedating patients for pain control slows down the number of procedures that can be done and decreases the billings for the physician, the hospital, and

---

[210] Arnold J. Sholder, MD: "Compassion is a lost art in today's health-care system." *Pittsburg Post-Gazette.* Wednesday, November 5, 1997.

the pathologist. It also costs the insurance company more. It's also true that Hank would be glad to pay more to get sedation, but he is not in control of the money.

Hank undergoes screaming agony during his biopsy, because the needs of the doctor, hospital, and insurance company all come before his needs. He was not even told about the ability to have "prostate blocks," shots that numb the prostate, making the procedure much more bearable for some men.

The Problem

Right now third parties are the most powerful entities in the health-care system.

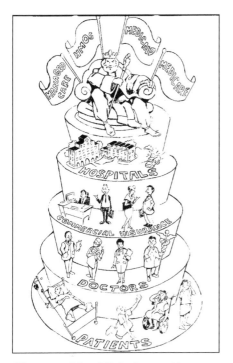

Figure 23. Third parties such as managed care, HMOs, Medicaid and Medicare sit atop the power structure in our health-care system. Patients are at the very bottom. (Artist: Ramie Balbuena)

In the examples mentioned above, HMOs, Insurance Companies, Medicare, Medicaid, Socialized Health Care, Hospitals, committees, and other entities made decisions for the patient. The patient has been stripped of power; patients are the weakest people in the health-care system.

We need to change the system so that the patient is the most powerful person in the health-care system. The second most powerful person should be the doctor. Only after this "team" should come the HMOs, insurance companies, Medicare, and Medicaid.

In the past, it was considered appropriate for doctors and committees to make decisions for patients. This was because patients did not have any medical information; they could not make an informed decision. But the Internet has changed all that. Today, patients often know more than doctors. Today, patients can make medical decisions for themselves, but they are not allowed to.

We all send our money off to HMOs, insurance companies, and to the government. Our health-care is then rationed back to us, not based on what we want, but based on what some third party wants. This is a horrible breakdown of free choice for patients. The patient should reign supreme!

Patients must keep control of the money, instead of relinquishing it to third parties, who could care less about individual needs. Third parties will never be competent to know an individual's needs.

One solution is Health Savings Accounts (also called Medical Savings Accounts). If set up properly, Health Savings Accounts (HSAs) are tax-free savings accounts from which patients pay for their medical care, pay for their catastrophic health-care insurance, and pay for their disability insurance. HSAs would be considered property that could be passed from parents to children.

With HSAs patients would have the power, they would call the shots, and health-care would dramatically improve. Costs would decrease, because a properly implemented HSA system would require that all health-care providers disclose prices before service is given. Patients would no longer be surprised three months later when they get their bill. We could actually shop for health-care like we do for computers! Prices would keep coming down, technology would keep getting better, and patients would get what they want.

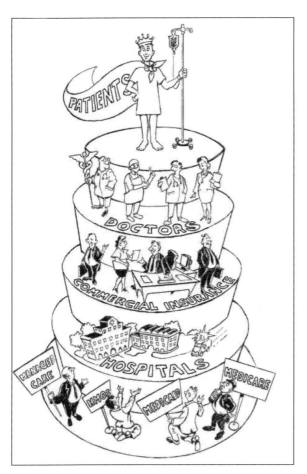

Figure 24. Patients should sit atop the power structure in the health-care system. (Artist: Ramie Balbuena)

People tell me that trying to change the health-care system is impossible. It has to start somewhere. The concept is simple. The most powerful person in healthcare needs to be you, the patient. The way for you to be most powerful is to control the money. I merely propose that patients control the money, and therefore their health!

Let's put patients back on top. Thank you.

Recommended Web Sites

SurvivingProstateCancerWithoutSurgery.org
ProstatitisAndBPH.org
EpididymitisFoundation.org
EjaculatoryDuctObstruction.org
VasectomyFoundation.org
VasectomyReversalFoundation.org
VaricoceleFoundation.org
PeyroniesFoundation.org
Orchitis.org
PhimosisFoundation.org
HerniaFoundation.org
Urethritis.org
Prostatitis.org
ProstateBooks.com
StemCellSociety.org
RosevilleBooks.com
Hennenfent.com

Acknowledgements

I started this book in 1984 and it was completed nearly 20 years later. I'm proud of the fact that I tracked down and interviewed many of the best urologists, oncologists, radiologists, infectious disease experts, epidemiologists, and statisticians in the world, and I cannot possibly acknowledge everyone to whom I am indebted, yet, I will thank as many as I can.

The reader must realize; however, that being listed here does not necessarily mean that the person endorses this book.

I want to thank agent Albert Zuckerman of Writer's House for suggesting the title and for being supportive. I thank Kent Henderson for the artwork and design of the front and back covers.

I thank all the men with prostate cancer who talked to me in person, by telephone, or by e-mail. Whenever possible, I quoted patients directly with their written permission. However, to protect medical privacy, composite characters were used if the same story was told over and over again by different men.

Editors

I wish to thank the many editors and writers who helped me with this book. I thank: Jack Handler (may he rest in peace), Albert LaFarge, Chris Roerden, Fred Powledge, Constance Cook, Hillel Black, Skip Press, Tom Ranieri, Carol Carter, Dale Evva Gelfand, Tari Parr, Norman Bauman, John Michel, Fred Feldman, H.L. "Budd" Lucus, Perry Gamsby, and Matt Kelley (who did some "ghostwriting"). I'd like to thank members of the Monmouth Writer's & Editor's Club, especially Dick Speer, Peggy Kulczewski, Sherri Ault, Jan Speer, and Tom Peterson.

The above people edited the grammatically perfect sections, while I no doubt wrote, or rewrote, the imperfect parts.

I also thank Mike DiFuccia and Karen Gillen at the Buchanan Center for the Arts, and I thank Dr. David Wise, author of *A Headache in the Pelvis*.

Organizations

I want to thank the Patient Advocates for Advanced Cancer Treatments (PAACT), Us TOO International, Man to Man, the American Prostate Society, the American Cancer Society, Americans for Free Choice in Medicine, the Prostatitis Foundation, the National Cancer Institute, the National Institutes of Health, the National Prostate Cancer Coalition, QuackWatch, the Prostate Cancer Charity, the Education Center for Prostate Cancer Patients, the National Center for Health Statistics, the People's Medical Society, the Galen Institute, and the Mellinger Foundation.

Leaders

Thanks to Lloyd Ney of PAACT; James Lewis, Jr., PhD, of the Education Center for Prostate Cancer Patients; Claude Gerard of the American Prostate Society; Hank Porterfield of the Alliance for Prostate Cancer Prevention; John Page and Bill Mulac of Us TOO International; and Jon Bernardes of the Prostate Help Association in England.

I want to thank Ken Smith, the long-time, outstanding volunteer webmaster for the Prostatitis Foundation. I thank Ron Henry; Jerry Lester, PhD; and Jim Sniechowski of the Men's Health Network. I thank E. Loren Buhle, Jr., PhD, the creator of OncoLink.

Thanks to Mike Hennenfent, President of the Prostatitis Foundation, for his tireless efforts and astonishing success in bringing the most common and most neglected prostate disease into the limelight.

I thank Peter Joseph, Dick Kerr, Jack Turley, Tony Stacier, Hugh Whitfield, Mike Sussman, Penny Allen, Bud Irish, Marvin Blumberg, Gary Huckaby, Bard Lindeman, Dave Trissel, Arthur Brown, Bill Cusack, Bettye L. Spatafora, Tom Feeney, and Jerry Bostick. Thanks to Hi Markham and Virgil H. Simons.

Thanks to Ed Price, Ralph Valle, Marriane Brosseau, and Bill Jenkins, Ed Piepmeier, Bob Southard, Don Swirnow, Richard Trax, Nancy Peress, Scott Barker, Linda Bridges, and Steve Corman, and others who have served to help men with prostate cancer.

Thanks to Alan Cocks, Engineer and Physicist, for his help on and off the Internet in promoting prostate health.

Physicians and Researchers

I want to thank all the physicians and researchers who allowed me to interview them by e-mail, phone, or in person. Many are mentioned within the book but I also acknowledge them here. I thank Timothy Wilt, MD, the director of the PIVOT trial (a prostate cancer study) at the Minneapolis Veterans Affairs Medical Center; family practitioner Steven H. Woolf, MD, writer of many excellent papers on prostate cancer; Otis Brawley, MD, a prostate cancer researcher at the National Cancer Institute, whose interview on television led me to look again at prostate cancer statistics; Jan-Erik Johansson, MD; Edward Vega, MD (may he rest in peace); and John Polacheck, MD, founder of the Tucson Prostatitis Center.

I thank Antonio Espinosa Feliciano Jr., MD; Noel de Vera, MD; Bienvenido S. Garcia, MD; and Anthony F. Cortez, MD; of the Manila Genitourinary Clinic. I thank Alfred Lazarte, MD, of the Cebu branch of the Manila Genitourinary Clinic.

I thank Ham Williams, MD; Gary Onik, MD; Donald Gleason, MD; Israel Barkin, MD; Duke Bahn, MD; Bob Werman, MD; Ronald Wheeler, MD; Fernand Labrie, MD, PhD; W. Reid Pitts, MD, FACS; Grigory Korik, MD, PhD (may he rest in peace); John Krieger, MD; Donald Riley, PhD; Jonas Muntzing, PhD; Gerald Domingue, PhD; and John Baust PhD, a cryoscience expert. Thanks to Steve Strum, MD, and Mark Scholz, MD, for their expertise, which they share with patients over the Internet. Thanks to Karen D. Godette, MD, a radiation oncologist who helps with a prostate cancer support group in Georgia. Thanks to Dr. Michael J. Zelefsky, a radiation oncologist; Jonathan Oppenheimer, MD, for his invaluable pathology advice; oncologist Robert Leibowitz, MD; urologist Haakon Ragde, MD; radiation oncologist Miljenko V. Pilepich, MD; radiation oncologist Dr. David Beyer; Dr. Howard Sandler; and Obstetrician-Gynecologist Fulton Saier, MD.

Attendings

I'd like to thank an outstanding group of attendings and teachers. I thank Harold Jayne, MD; Gary Strange, MD; David Howes, MD; Helene Connolly, MD; Carl Ferraro, MD; Mary Ann Cooper, MD; Tim Turnbull, MD; Liz Orsay, MD; Yogi Viggaria, MD; Ron Barreca, MD; Douglas Propp, MD; Mary Ann Cooper, MD; John L. Zautcke, MD; Ron Tanaway, MD; Kris Narasimhan, MD; Don Steiner, MD; Harold Chin, MD; Song-Ling Chang, MD; Dr. Mustafa; Richard Feldman, MD; George Hossfeld, MD; Tim Rittenberry, MD; Max Koenigsberg, MD; Ron Lee, MD (may he rest in peace); Dennis Uehara, MD; Herb Sutherland, DO; and Jane Caseley, MD. If I forgot anyone, it was by accident.

Residency

I thank a group of outstanding classmates who taught me so many intangibles: Jeff Schwartz, MD; Mark Kling, MD; Tess Hogan, MD; Dana Perry, MD; Edward Sloan, MD; Robert Zalinski, MD; Charles Ford, MD; Ray Hart, MD; Mark Langdorf, MD; Dave Halperin, MD; and Karen Chermel, MD. I offer special thanks to Deborah Weber, MD, who interested me in medical writing and editing.

Statisticians

I want to thank the following people who have special expertise in medical statistics: Clark Hickman, PhD, a statistician and research methodologist; Donald K. Corle; David Eddy, MD, PhD; Craig Fleming; Grace L. Lu-Yao, MD; John Wennberg, MD; Janet Stanford, PhD; Brent Blumenstein, PhD; Mithat Gonen, PhD; Melinda Drum, PhD; Reinhold Bergstrom, PhD; and George Conklin, PhD.

Reporters

Thanks to Susan Powter, who spent time on her radio show talking about prostate cancer; Gabe Mirkin, MD, who has written about prostate cancer and prostatitis; Timothy Johnson, MD, who has spoken about both prostate cancer and Prostatitis; and to Isadore Rosenfeld, MD, who has written about prostatitis in Parade Magazine.

Thanks to Andy Grove, Chairman of Intel, who wrote an article about his own prostate cancer in FORTUNE Magazine, and to Ed DeHart who wrote an article about his own prostate cancer in UROLOGY.

Economists

I'd like to thank economists Robert Eisner, John C. Goodman, Gerald Musgrave, and all the economics professors at Northwestern University.

Others

I thank Jim Johnson, MD; Bob Williams, MD; and Donza Warden, MD.

I thank Hetzal Hartley, MD; Anthony Marks, MD; Dan Icenogle, MD; Richard Icenogle, MD (may he rest in peace); Paulette Wilson, MD; Dave Wright, MD; Mark Marshall, MD; and Tom Preddy, MD.

I want to thank David Strickler, and my elementary school teachers and high school teachers, for making science, math, and English spectacular in a small town. I thank Russell Lober (may he rest in peace). I thank the faculty of the University of Illinois Medical School and of the University of Illinois Affiliated Hospitals Emergency Medicine Program.

I'd like to thank Joe Simonson, Mark Boulware, Chuck Grant, Steve Gibbs, Tim Ingles, Donnie Johnson, Danny Thomas, Mike Huston, Dan Pettinger, Howard Rescot, Brian Elliott, Terry Davis, Pam Livermore, Kevin Horath, Brad McCullough, Ronnie Bowers, Rick Horney, Freddy Langford, Mike Taylor, Ken Klein, Charlie Mehler, JD Freedman, Jeffrey P. Burds, Howard Price and Keli'i Akina. I thank my parents, Mike and Betty Hennenfent, and my siblings George, Frank, Nick, Nancy, and Steve.

Lastly, I thank the creators of the Palm Pilot.

About the Artists

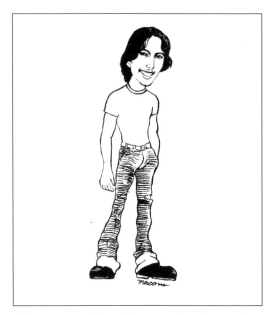

Figure 25. Jun Macam by Jun Macam.

Jun Macam is a dancer by profession and a part-time freelance illustrator. He has illustrated books and comics, and has also done industrial product design. While working on this book Jun was astonished about how often men would ask him about prostate disease, and was surprised to realize how uniformed men were about the prostate.

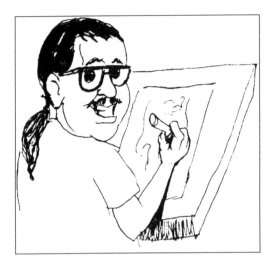

Figure 26. Dave Curbis by Dave Curbis

Dave Curbis is a self-taught artist, cartoonist, and portrait artist. He has done promotional work for a local hospital, and as a freelance artist has done work ranging from T-shirts to garage doors. He is aware of the use of the transurethral resection of the prostate (TURP) on many men with various prostatic complaints, and remains dismayed that alternative therapies are not being offered.

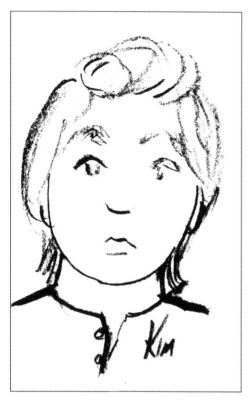

Figure 27. Mike Kim by Mike Kim.

Mike Kim is a practicing freelance writer and cartoonist whose work has appeared in many consumer and trade magazines such as *Modern Medicine, Physician's Management, New Women, Saturday Review, Bulletin of The Atomic Scientists, Writer's Digest*, etc., as well as many educational and commercial textbooks in the computer and educational fields.

About the Author

Bradley Hennenfent, MD, is a graduate of Northwestern University, the University of Illinois Medical School, and the University of Illinois Affiliated Hospitals Emergency Medicine Residency Program.

He first became interested in the prostate when his Uncle Steve, who inspired him to attend medical school, died from his prostate cancer treatment in 1984.

As Dr. Hennenfent researched the prostate, he became increasingly dismayed by the drastic operations that men were being subjected to without an understanding of their consequences. He discovered that the methods of diagnosis and treatment of prostate cancer were controversial, and that the research published by urologists is substantially flawed.

Dr. Hennenfent became a men's health activist. He began doing original research. He founded the Internet newsgroups sci.med.prostate.cancer, sci.med.prostate.bph, and sci.med.prostate.prostatitis. He was also one of the original founders of the Internet *Prostate Problems Mailing List*. Together with his father, Mike Hennenfent, he co-founded the nonprofit Prostatitis Foundation (www.prostatitis.org), where almost a million men per year visit for help.

Dr. Hennenfent has been published in the *British Journal of Urology*, the *Digital Urology Journal, Emerging Infectious Diseases, Annals of Emergency Medicine, Consultant*, EMERGINDEX, *Techniques in Urology*, and the *Journal of Pelvic Surgery*. He also authored a monograph entitled the *Prostatitis Syndromes*, donating all proceeds to the non-profit Prostatitis Foundation.

Besides being a physician, Dr. Hennenfent is also an economist who believes that a well-designed health-care system is more important to the health of a nation's people than any single physician's skill and knowledge. He has traveled the world doing medical research and studying health-care delivery systems.

Dr. Hennenfent has delivered more than forty-five lectures at various hospitals. He owns a patent that enables less painful digital rectal examinations and prostatic massage.

Dr. Hennenfent has spent time educating congress on the need for prostatitis research and has helped secure millions of dollars in federal funding for prostatitis research.

Among the author's heroes are Jessica Mitford, whose book, *The American Way of Death*, exposed the funeral industry's financial exploitation of grieving relatives; Randy Shiltz, whose book, *And the Band Played On*, exposed the system's lack of response to the AIDS epidemic; and Hillary Johnson, author of *Osler's Web: Inside the Chronic Fatigue Syndrome Epidemic*, which exposed another shameful response of the medical system to a major health issue.

Dr. Hennenfent is a fan of *Lies, Damn Lies, and Statistics: The Manipulation of Public Opinion in America*, the book by Michael Wheeler that first brought popular attention to how and why statistics are often misused; the hilarious *How to Lie with Statistics* by Darrell Huff; and *The Honest Truth about Lying with Statistics* by Cooper B. Holmes.

Dr. Hennenfent lives in downstate, Illinois where he writes, does medical research, and contributes to the non-profit Prostatitis Foundation. Someday, he hopes to open a clinical research center for prostate diseases and to organize a biomedical company to do research.

Dr. Hennenfent started the web sites: SurvivingProstateCancerWithoutSurgery.org, ProstatitisAndBPH.org, and EpididymitisFoundation.org.

To contact Dr. Hennenfent about medical information, please post to the message boards on one of his web sites. To suggest changes in this book, please send e-mail to Dr.Hennenfent@gmail.com.

How to Order More Books

Order online at:
Amazon.com
SurvivingProstateCancerWithoutSurgery.org
RosevilleBooks.com

Roseville Books
www.RosevilleBooks.com
E-mail: Roseville.Books@gmail.com
Tel. 206-350-1242
Fax: 206-350-1242

To comment on this book, send e-mail to:
Dr.Hennenfent@gmail.com.

For the latest news about the book, and for online discussion, visit:
SurvivingProstateCancerWithoutSurgery.org.

This book is currently available online at:
Amazon.com

Figure Index

Index

Made in the USA
San Bernardino, CA
24 April 2013